ABC OF HYPERTENSION

Fifth Edition

Edited by

D GARETH BEEVERS
Professor of medicine, University Department of Medicine,
City Hospital, Birmingham

GREGORY Y H LIP
Professor of cardiovascular medicine, University Department of Medicine,
City Hospital, Birmingham

and

EOIN O'BRIEN
Professor of molecular pharmacology, Conway Institute of Biomolecular and
Biomedical Research, University College Dublin, Belfield, Dublin 4, Ireland

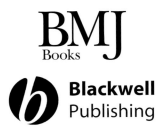

BMJ
Books

Blackwell
Publishing

© 1981, 1987, 1995, 2001 BMJ Books
© 2007 Blackwell Publishing Ltd
BMJ Books is an imprint of the BMJ Publishing Group Limited, used under licence

Blackwell Publishing Inc., 350 Main Street, Malden, Massachuesetts 02148-5020, USA
Blackwell Publishing Ltd, 9600 Garsington Road, Oxford OX4 2DQ, UK
Blackwell Publishing Asia Pty Ltd, 550 Swanston Street, Carlton, Victoria 3053, Australia

First published 1981
Second edition 1987
Third edition 1995
Fourth edition 2001
Fifth edition 2007

1 2007

Library of Congress Cataloging-in-Publication Data
Beevers, D. G. (D. Gareth)
    ABC of hypertension / D. Gareth Beevers, Gregory Y. H. Lip, and Eoin O'Brien.—5th ed.
        p. ; cm.
    Includes bibliographical references and index.
    ISBN: 978-1-4051-3061-5 (alk. paper)
    1. Hypertension. I. Lip, Gregory Y. H. II. O'Brien, Eoin. III. Title.
    [DNLM: 1. Hypertension—diagnosis. 2. Blood Pressure Determination—methods.
3. Hypertension—therapy.   WG 340 B415a 2007]
    RC685. H8B34 2007
    616.1′32—dc22

                                                                2006027936

ISBN: 978-1-4051-3061-5

A catalogue record for this title is available from the British Library

Cover image is courtesy of TEK Image/Science Photo Library

Set in 9/11 pts New Baskerville by Newgen Imaging Systems (P) Ltd, Chennai, India
Printed and bound in Singapore by Markono Print Media Pte Ltd

Commissioning Editor: Eleanor Lines
Development Editors: Sally Carter, Nick Morgan
Editorial Assistant: Victoria Pittman
Production Controller: Rachel Edwards

For further information on Blackwell Publishing, visit our website:
http://www.blackwellpublishing.com

Contents

Preface

The first edition of the *ABC of Hypertension*, published in 1981, rose out of a series of review articles published in the *British Medical Journal* under the titles of *ABC of blood pressure measurement* and *ABC of blood pressure reduction*. Since that time there have been a great many advances in our understanding of clinical aspects of hypertension that have necessitated regular updating. In particular there have been major improvements in the measurement of blood pressure with increasing awareness of the relative importance of 24 hour ambulatory blood pressure monitoring versus casual office blood pressure readings. In addition, the focus of the management of hypertensive patients has moved to encompass a measure of total cardiovascular risk rather than just the blood pressure. This has been helped by the ready availability of simple risk charts, particularly those published by the British Hypertension Society and the joint British Societies. Along with this there has been an increasing awareness that the height for systolic blood pressure is a better predictor of cardiovascular risk than the diastolic blood pressure and that isolated systolic hypertension, with its high risk, is well worth treating. Even today, however, many clinicians who were originally taught that the diastolic pressure was more important than the systolic are finding this radical change in emphasis to be somewhat startling.

The first edition of the *ABC of Hypertension* was published before the era of angiotensin converting enzyme inhibitors. There is no doubt that these agents, together with the more recently synthesised angiotensin receptor blockers are by far the most tolerable antihypertensive drugs. They have transformed the treatment of diabetic hypertensives and hypertensives with concomitant heart disease or nephropathy. Since the publication of the fourth edition of the *ABC of Hypertension*, we have seen publication of the Losartan Intervention For Endpoint (LIFE) study and the Anglo Scandinavian Cardiac Outcomes Trial (ASCOT). In both of these trials the drugs that block the renin-angiotensin system were found to be superior to previous standard regimes of atenolol with or without a thiazide diuretic. These two trials have heralded the end of the supremacy of β blockers in the treatment of uncomplicated hypertension. Again, this will be a radical turnaround for those clinicians who have put their faith in β blockers for uncomplicated essential hypertension in the hope that they might be better at preventing first coronary events than other agents.

Thus, since 1980 we have become better at assessing our patients' blood pressure, better at assessing their cardiovascular risk, and we have more effective and more tolerable antihypertensive agents. In previous years a clinician, when faced with a patient where the value of treatment was open to question, might have taken the view "when in doubt, don't treat." Nowadays the same clinician, when faced with a similar patient, is more likely to say "when in doubt, treat." This view, together with the arrival of the statins, means that lives are being saved and people are living longer.

Publication of the LIFE trial and ASCOT brings us to a sort of plateau in the topic of clinical hypertension research. Although there is no doubt that there are many advances to be looked forward to in the topic of the basic cardiovascular sciences, it is unlikely that we will have much more information on clinical care for a few years. Perhaps the biggest problem now is to improve the quality and efficiency of the delivery of the various validated treatments to individual patients. We are acutely aware that this healthcare delivery is mainly the responsibility of the primary healthcare team based in general practice. We hope that this fifth edition of the *ABC of Hypertension* provides sufficient evidence based material to guide clinicians in the correct manner of investigating and managing hypertensive patients while providing pragmatic guidance on good clinical practice that can be applied in any healthcare delivery system. Things have changed so much over the last 25 years that the *ABC of Hypertension* remains necessary to help clinicians manage the most common chronic medical condition world-wide. We hope therefore that this edition will provide useful guidance for clinicians in developing as well as developed countries.

DG Beevers
GYH Lip
E O'Brien

1 Prevalence and causes

G Y H Lip, D G Beevers

In the population, blood pressure is a continuous, normally distributed variable. No separate subgroups of people with and without hypertension exist. A consistent continuous gradient exists between usual levels of blood pressure and the risk of coronary heart disease and stroke, and this gradient continues down to blood pressures that are well below the average for the population. This means that much of the burden of renal disease and cardiovascular disease related to blood pressure can be attributed to blood pressures within the so called "normotensive" or average range for Western populations.

The main concern for doctors is what level of blood pressure needs drug treatment. The pragmatic definition of hypertension is the level of blood pressure at which treatment is worthwhile. This level varies from patient to patient and balances the risks of untreated hypertension in different types of patients and the known benefits of reducing blood pressure, while taking into account the disadvantages of taking drugs and the likelihood of side effects.

> **"In an operational sense, hypertension should be defined in terms of a blood pressure level above which investigation and treatment do more good than harm" Grimley Evans J, Rose G. Br Med Bull 1971;27:37–42**

Systolic blood pressure has a strong tendency to increase with advancing age, so the prevalence of hypertension (and its complications) also increases with age. Hypertension thus is as much a disorder of populations as of individual people. Globally, high blood pressure accounts for more deaths than many common conditions and is a major burden of disease.

As hypertension is the most important risk factor for cardiovascular disease, achievement of a universal target systolic blood pressure of 140 mm Hg should produce a reduction of 28–44% in the incidence of stroke and 20–35% of coronary heart disease. This could prevent about 21 400 deaths from stroke and 41 400 deaths from coronary heart disease in the United Kingdom each year. It would also mean about 42 800 fewer fatal and non-fatal strokes and 82 800 fewer coronary heart disease events per year in the United Kingdom alone. Globally, as hypertension is becoming more common, coronary heart disease and stroke correspondingly are becoming common, particularly in developing countries.

A recently published analysis of pooled data from different regions of the world estimated the overall prevalence and absolute burden of hypertension in 2000 and the global burden in 2025. Overall, 26.4% of the adult population in 2000 had hypertension and 29.2% were projected to have this condition by 2025. The estimated total number of adults with hypertension in 2000 was 972 million: 333 million in economically developed countries and 639 million in economically developing countries. The number of adults with hypertension in 2025 thus is predicted to increase by about 60% to a total of 156 billion.

The development of hypertension reflects a complex and dynamic interaction between genetic and environmental factors. In some primitive communities in which obesity is rare and salt intake is low, hypertension is virtually unknown, and blood pressure does not increase with advancing age.

Studies have investigated Japanese people migrating from Japan to the west coast of America. In Japan, high blood

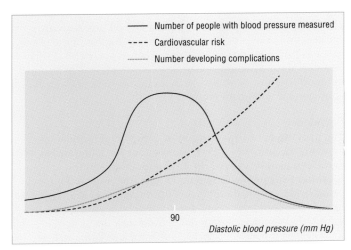

Hypertension: a disease of quantity not quality

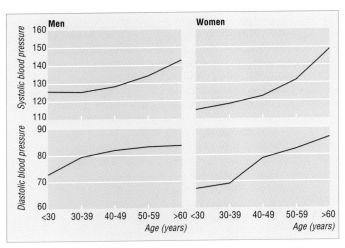

Birmingham Factory Screening Project (figure excludes data from 165 patients on drugs that lower blood pressure). Adapted from Lane D, et al. *J Human Hypertens* 2002;16:267–73

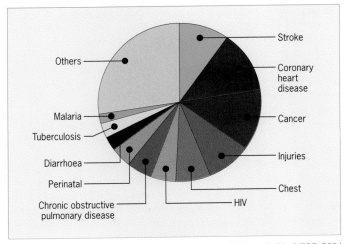

Worldwide causes of death. Adapted from Mackay J, Mensah GA, WHO 2004

pressure is common and the incidence of stroke is high, but coronary heart disease is rare. When Japanese people moved across the Pacific Ocean, a reduction in the incidence of hypertension and stroke was seen, but the incidence of coronary heart disease increased. These studies strongly suggest that, although racial differences exist in the predisposition to hypertension, environmental factors still play a significant role. The United Kingdom also has a pronounced north–south gradient in blood pressure, with pressures higher in the north of the country. Studies that compare urban and rural populations in African populations also show clear differences in blood pressure between urban and rural societies with the same genetic composition.

Prevalence

The prevalence of hypertension in the general population depends on the arbitrary criteria used for its definition, as well as the population studied. In 2853 participants in the Birmingham Factory Screening Project, the odds ratios for being hypertensive after adjustment for age were 1.56 and 2.40 for African-Caribbean men and women, respectively, and 1.31 for South-Asian men compared with Europeans.

The Third National Health and Nutrition Examination Survey 1988–91 (NHANES III) showed that 24% of the adult population in the United States, which represents more than 43 million people, have hypertension (>140/90 mm Hg or current treatment for hypertension). The prevalence of hypertension varies from 4% in people aged 18–29 years to 65% in people older than 80 years. Prevalence is higher among men than women, and the prevalence in African-Americans is higher than in Caucasians and Mexican-Americans (32.4%, 23.3%, and 22.6%, respectively). Most cases of hypertension in young adults result from increases in diastolic blood pressure, whereas in elderly people, isolated increases in systolic blood pressure are more common and account for 60% of cases of hypertension in men and 70% in women. Hypertension generally affects ≤10% of the population up to the age of 34 years. By the age of 65, however, more than half of the population has hypertension.

Incidence

Unfortunately, few data are available on the incidence of new onset hypertension. The incidence of hypertension does increase sharply with age, with higher rates in men.

Follow up of people in the Framingham Heart Study after 30 years found that the two year incidence of new onset hypertension increases from 3.3% in men and 1.5% in women aged 30–39 years to 6.2% in men and 8.6% in women aged 70–79 years. People with "high normal" blood pressure at first examination were at greater risk of developing sustained hypertension over the ensuing years. Some authorities argue that high normal blood pressure should be reclassified as "prehypertensive."

"High normal" blood pressure is one of the strongest predictors for the later development of hypertension. At the individual level, however, blood pressure in childhood is poorly predictive of later levels of blood pressure or the risk of hypertension.

Age

In western societies, blood pressure rises with increasing age, and people with high baseline blood pressures have a faster increase than those with normal or below average pressures. In rural non-Westernised societies, however, hypertension is rare, and the increase in pressure with age is much smaller. The level of blood pressure accurately predicts coronary heart disease and stroke at all ages, although in very elderly people, the

Prevalence of hypertension (>160/95 mm Hg or treated) in the Birmingham Factory Screening Project

Population	Men (%)	Women (%)
African-Caribbean	30.8	34.4
European	19.4	12.9
South Asian	16.0	–

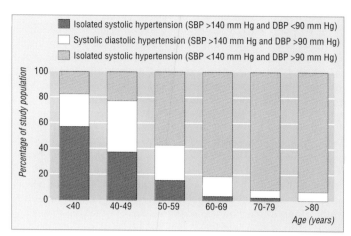

Hypertension subtypes from the NHANES III study (DBP = diastolic blood pressure, SBP = systolic blood pressure). Adapted from Franklin SS, et al. *Hypertension* 2001;37:869–74

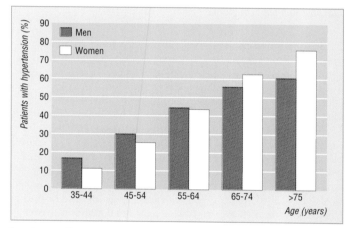

Prevalence of hypertension in US citizens aged ≥35 years by age and sex in the NHANES III study (1988–94). Those classified as having hypertension had a systolic blood pressure ≥140 mm Hg or a diastolic blood pressure of ≥90 mm Hg, were taking antihypertensive drugs. Adapted from Wolz M, et al. *Am J Hypertens* 2000;13:104–4

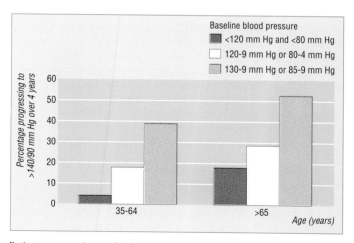

Patients progressing to develop new hypertension in the Framingham Heart Study. Adapted from Vasan RS, et al. *Lancet* 2001;358:1682–6

relation is less clear. This may be because many people with increased blood pressures have died and those with lower pressure may have subclinical or overt heart disease that causes their blood pressure to decrease.

Ethnic origin

People of African origin have been studied well in North America, but whether these data can be fully applicable to the African-Caribbean populations in the United Kingdom or similar populations in Africa or the West Indies is uncertain. All studies of people of African origin from urban communities, however, show a higher prevalence than in Caucasian people. Yet hypertension is rare in black people who live in rural Africa. Whether any particular level of blood pressure carries a worse prognosis in people of African origin or whether survival is much the same as in people of European origin but with more strokes and fewer heart attacks is uncertain.

Even when correction is made for obesity, socioeconomic, and dietary factors, ethnic factors remain in the predisposition to hypertension. These differences are probably related to ethnic differences in salt sensitivity. There is little evidence to show that people of African origin in the United Kingdom and United States consume more salt than people of European origin. There is evidence that salt loading raises blood pressure more in people of African origin and that salt restriction is more beneficial. These differences in salt sensitivity may also be related to the finding that plasma levels of renin and angiotensin in African-American people are about half those in Americans of European origin. As discussed later, differences in renin may explain ethnic differences in responses to antihypertensive drugs.

Sex

Before the age of about 50 years, hypertension is less common in women than men. After this age, blood pressure in women gradually increases to about the same level as in men. Consequently, the complications of hypertension are less common in younger women. This protection may be related to beneficial effects of oestrogens or a harmful effect of androgens on vascular risk.

Increasing evidence shows that women with a past history of pre-eclampsia and pregnancy induced or gestational hypertension have an increased risk of hypertension and cardiovascular disease in later life. Such women should be considered to be at higher risk and need regular monitoring.

Causes of hypertension

In around 5% of people with hypertension, the high blood pressure is explained by underlying renal or adrenal diseases. In the remaining 95%, no clear cause can be identified. Such cases of hypertension are described as "essential" or "primary" hypertension. Essential hypertension is related to the interplay of genetic and environmental factors, but the precise role of these is uncertain.

Environmental and lifestyle causes of hypertension

Salt

Salt intake has a consistent and direct effect on blood pressure. As stated earlier, migration studies in African and Japanese people have shown changes in blood pressure when moving from one environmental background to another. The factor most likely to be involved is a change in salt intake.

Many potential mechanisms for how salt causes hypertension have been suggested. Evidence from observational

---

Blood pressure in populations of African origin in the United Kingdom: review of 14 adult cross sectional studies in 1978

Blood pressure	Men	Women
Systolic higher than Europeans	10 of 14	10 of 12
Diastolic higher than Europeans	11 of 14	10 of 12
Hypertension more common	8 of 10	8 of 9

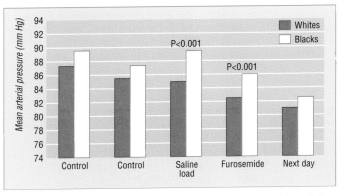

Effect of salt loading in black and white normotensive people. Adapted from Luft FC, et al. *Circulation* 1979;59:643–50

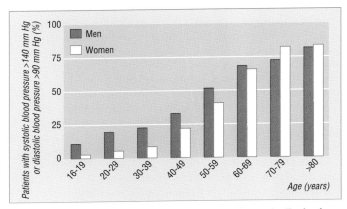

Prevalence of secondary hypertension in the Health Survey for England 1998. Adapted from Primatesta P, et al. *Hypertension* 2001;38:827–32

Prevalence of secondary hypertension in three published surveys

Type of hypertension	Study		
	Rudnick, 1977	Sinclair, 1987	Anderson, 1994
Essential hypertension	94.0%	92.1%	89.5%
Renal disease	5.0%	5.6%	1.8%
Renal artery disease	0.2%	0.7%	3.3%
Cushing's syndrome	0.2%	0.1%	–
Oral contraceptives	0.2%	1.0%	–
Phaeochromocytoma	–	0.1%	0.3%
Coarctation	0.2%	–	–

How does salt cause hypertension?

- Increased circulating fluid volume
- Inappropriate sodium:renin ratio, with failure of renin to suppress increased intracellular sodium
- Waterlogged, swollen endothelial cells that reduce the interior diameter of arterioles
- Permissive rise in intracellular calcium, which leads to contraction of vascular smooth muscle

epidemiological studies, animal models, and randomised controlled trials in patients with hypertension and normal blood pressure all point to a causal relation between salt and blood pressure. The potential clinical and public health impact of relatively modest salt restriction thus is substantial.

The Intersalt project, which involved more than 10 000 men and women aged 20–59 years in 52 different populations in 32 countries, quite clearly showed that the increase in blood pressure with advancing age in urban societies was related to the amount of salt in the diet. Positive associations between urinary excretion of sodium (a marker of salt intake) and blood pressure were observed within and between populations. In men and women of all ages, an increase in sodium intake of 100 mmol/day was estimated to be associated with an average increase in systolic blood pressure of up to 6 mm Hg. The association was larger for older people.

This finding was supported by a meta-analysis of the many individual population surveys of blood pressure in relation to salt intake. Law et al performed a meta-analysis of 78 trials of the effect of sodium intake on blood pressure and reported that a reduction in daily salt intake of about 3 g (attainable by moderate reductions in dietary intake of salt) in people aged 50–59 years should lower systolic blood pressure by an average of 5 mm Hg. An average reduction in blood pressure of this magnitude in the general population of most Western countries would reduce the incidence of stroke by 25% and the incidence of ischaemic heart disease by 15%.

A number of clinical trials also show reductions in blood pressure after restriction of salt intake (see chapter 8). In a recent study in the United Kingdom, a reduction in daily salt intake from 10 g to 5 g over one month in a group of men and women aged 60–78 years with hypertension resulted in an average fall in systolic blood pressure of 7 mm Hg.

The value of the restriction of salt intake in people without hypertension is more controversial. Data pooled from the limited studies available suggest that reduction of salt intake to about 6 g/day should reduce systolic blood pressure by about 2 mm Hg and diastolic pressure by 1 mm Hg. Although clinically unimportant, this reduction, if genuine and sustained, would be expected to bring about a 17% reduction in the prevalance of hypertension.

Potassium

The relation between intake of sodium, intake of potassium, and blood pressure is complex and has not been resolved completely. The effect of dietary intake of potassium on blood pressure is difficult to separate from that of salt.

The Intersalt project showed that high intake of potassium was associated with a lower prevalence of hypertension. Urinary sodium and potassium ratios in the United States showed marked differences between black and white people, despite little difference in their sodium intake or excretion. Dietary intake of potassium also has been related inversely to the risk of stroke. The antihypertensive effects of potassium chloride and other potassium salts are the same, which indicates that it is the potassium that matters. Most of the potassium in the diet is not in the form of potassium chloride but potassium citrate and potassium bicarbonate.

Calcium and magnesium

A weak inverse association exists between intake of calcium and blood pressure. Nonetheless, data from clinical trials of calcium supplementation on blood pressure are inconsistent, and the overall effect probably is minimal. A weak relation also exists between intake of magnesium and blood pressure, but the use of magnesium supplements has been disappointing.

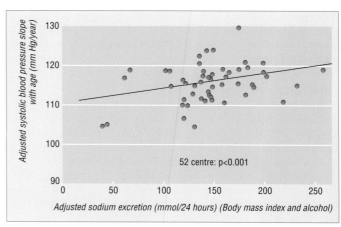

Intersalt project. Adapted from INTERSALT cooperative research group. *BMJ* 1988;297:319–28

INTERSALT project: sodium excretion and systolic blood pressure in individual centres

Variable	Adjusted for	
	Age, sex	Age, sex, body mass index (kg/m²), alcohol, and potassium
Centres with positive change	39	33
Centres with significantly positive change	15	8
Combined centre coefficient per mm Hg per 100 mmol of sodium	1.63*	1.00*
Combined centre coefficient corrected for reliability	3.54	2.17

*$P < 0.001$.
Adapted from INTERSALT cooperative research group. *BMJ* 1988;297:319–28

INTERSALT project: within centre coefficients for potassium in 24 hour urine sampling adjusted for age and sex

Variable	Blood pressure	
	Systolic	Diastolic
Positive coefficients:	24	29
Significant	0	2
Negative coefficients:	28	23
Significant	2	2
Centres	52	52

Adapted from INTERSALT cooperative research group. *BMJ* 1988;297:319–28

Weight

People who are obese or overweight tend to have higher blood pressures than thin people. Even after taking into account the confounding effects of obese arms and inappropriate cuff sizes on blood pressure measurement, a positive relation still exists between blood pressure and obesity—whether expressed as body mass index (weight (kg)/(height (m)^2)), relative weight, skinfold thickness, or waist to hip ratio. An increase in body weight from childhood to young adulthood is a major predictor of adult hypertension.

This association is clearly related to a high energy diet, although other dietary factors may be implicated (for example, high intake of sodium). The risk is greater in patients with truncal obesity, which may be a marker for insulin resistance, activation of the sympathetic nervous system, or other pathophysiological mechanisms that link obesity and hypertension. The close association of obesity with diabetes mellitus, insulin resistance, and impaired glucose tolerance and high levels of plasma lipids also partly explains why obesity is such a powerful risk factor for cardiovascular disease.

In general, trials of weight reduction show changes in mean systolic blood pressure and diastolic blood pressure of about 5.2 mm Hg in patients with hypertension and 2.5 mm Hg in people with normal blood pressure. This translates roughly to a reduction in blood pressure of 1 mm Hg for each kilogram of weight loss.

Alcohol

Epidemiological studies have shown a positive relation between alcohol consumption and blood pressure, which is independent of age, obesity, cigarette smoking, social class, and sodium excretion. In the British Regional Heart Study, about 10% of cases of hypertension (blood pressure ≥160/95 mm Hg) could be attributed to moderate or heavy drinking. Generally, the greater the alcohol consumption, the higher the blood pressure, although teetotallers seem to have slightly higher blood pressures than moderate drinkers.

The reversibility of hypertension related to alcohol has been shown in population surveys and alcohol loading and restriction studies. A reduction in weekly alcohol consumption is associated with clinically significant decreases in blood pressure, independent of weight loss, in people with normal blood pressure and those with hypertension. A reduction in intake of about three drinks per week was estimated to result in an average fall in supine systolic blood pressure of 3.1 mm Hg.

The mechanisms of the relation between alcohol and blood pressure are uncertain, but they are not explained by body mass index or salt intake. The effects of alcohol on blood pressure may include:

- A direct pressor effect of alcohol
- Sensitisation of resistance vessels to pressor substances
- Stimulation of the sympathetic nervous system (possibly as a result of fluctuating levels of alcohol in blood)
- Increased production of adrenocorticoid hormones.

Stress

Psychological or environmental stress may play a small part in the aetiology of hypertension, although studies frequently have been confounded by other environmental or lifestyle factors. Although research has focused on possible direct effects of psychosocial "stress" on blood pressure, "stressors" such as poverty, unemployment, and poor education are involved, as are other aspects of lifestyle that are linked to hypertension (including obesity, a diet high in salt, and physical inactivity).

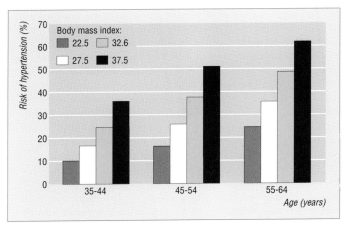

Hypertension and body mass index (BMI) observed in the NHANES III study. Adapted from Thompson PD, et al. *Arch Intern Med* 1999;159:2177–83

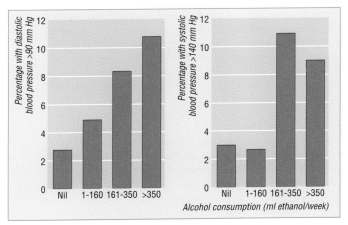

Alcohol and hypertension. in a working population. Adapted from Arkwright P, et al. *Circulation* 1982;66:60–6

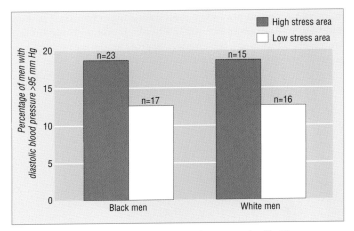

Stress, ethnicity, and hypertension in men. Stress was classified by residential area and crime rates. Adapted from Harburg E, et al. *J Chronic Dis* 1973;26:595–611

Although stressful stimuli may cause an acute rise in blood pressure, whether this has any significance in the long term is doubtful. A reduction in psychological stress through biofeedback techniques may reduce blood pressure in the clinic, although little effect on ambulatory blood pressure recordings at home is seen. In a recent meta-analysis of trials that involved stress management techniques such as meditation and biofeedback with at least six months of follow up, only eight trials that met the inclusion criteria were identified and the findings were inconsistent, with very small pooled falls in systolic and diastolic blood pressure (1.0/1.1 mm Hg).

Exercise

Blood pressure increases sharply during physical activity, but people who undertake regular exercise are fitter and healthier and have lower blood pressures. Such people, however, also may have a healthier diet and more sensible drinking and smoking habits.

Recent studies suggest an independent relation between increased levels of exercise and lower blood pressures; vigorous exercise might be harmful, but all other grades of exercise increasingly are beneficial. Observational epidemiological studies also show that physical activity reduces the risk of heart attack and stroke, which may be mediated by beneficial effects on blood pressure. In the British Regional Heart Study, an inverse association between physical activity and systolic and diastolic blood pressure was seen in men who did not have evidence of ischaemic heart disease. This association was independent of age, body mass index, social class, smoking status, total levels of cholesterol, and levels of high density lipoprotein cholesterol.

Other dietary factors

Blood pressure in vegetarians is generally lower than in non-vegetarians. Substitution of animal products with vegetable products reduces blood pressure. The mechanisms of this beneficial effect of a vegetarian diet are uncertain. It may, in part, be related to a lower intake of dairy products or salt. Alternatively the lower blood pressures may be related to a higher dietary intake of potassium, fibre, flavinoids, or vegetable protein (see Elliott P, et al. *Arch Intern Med* 2006;166:79–87).

Large amounts of omega 3 fatty acids from fish oils may reduce blood pressure in people with hypertension. In observational studies, important inverse associations of blood pressure with intake of fibre and protein have been reported.

Although caffeine acutely increases blood pressure, tolerance to this pressor effect is generally believed to develop rapidly. A recent report suggests an association of raised blood pressure with an excessive intake of cola drinks, with an effect seen with "diet" and high energy cola drinks. This may be related to their caffeine content.

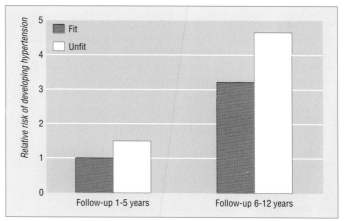

Physical fitness and later hypertension. Adapted from Blair SN, et al. *JAMA* 1984;252:487–90

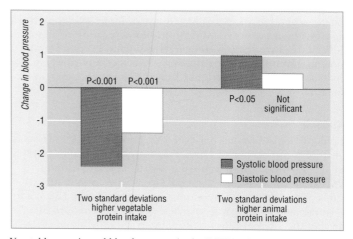

Vegetable protein and blood pressure in the INTERMAP study. Adapted from Elliot P, et al. *Arch Intern Med* 2006;166:79–87 and Stamler J, et al. *J Human Hypertens* 2003;17:591–608

The table of prevalence of hypertension is adapted from Lane D, et al. *J Human Hypertens* 2002;16:267–73. The table of blood pressure in populations of African origin in the UK is adapted from Agyemang C, Bhopal, RS. *J Human Hypertens* 2003;17:523–34. The table of secondary hypertension is adapted from Rudnick NR, et al. *CMAJ* 1977;117:492–7; Sinclair AM, et al. *Arch Intern Med* 1987;147:1289–93; and Anderson GH, et al. *J Hypertens* 1994;12:609–15.

2 Hypertension and vascular risk

G Y H Lip, D G Beevers

A close dose-response relation exists between the height of systolic and diastolic blood pressures and the risk of stroke or coronary heart disease. This effect is seen in all ages, both sexes, and all ethnic groups.

Malignant hypertension

Very high blood pressure that exceeds 200/120 mm Hg is relatively uncommon and affects only 0.5% of the adult population. Malignant, or malignant phase hypertension with retinal haemorrhages, exudates with or without papilloedema is even more rare, being seen in about three per 100 000 population. Malignant hypertension carries a very grave prognosis when untreated, with nearly 90% of patients dying within two years. Most patients die of renal failure, stroke, or left ventricular failure. With modern treatment, survival is much improved, with >80% of patients surviving five years.

Early detection and management of mild grades of hypertension means that malignant hypertension is declining in incidence. Often no underlying cause of the increased blood pressure is identifiable, but intrinsic renal disease is seen more often in patients with malignant hypertension than in those with non-malignant hypertension.

Blood pressure and risk

The close relation between the height of the blood pressure and the risk of heart attack and stroke continues down to pressures that are average or even less than the average for the general population. This means that people with systolic blood pressures as low as 130 mm Hg are at greater risk than those with even lower pressures. In the absence of concomitant unrelated diseases (such as cancer) or pre-existing cardiovascular damage (such as after myocardial infarction), low systolic and diastolic pressures are not associated with increased mortality or morbidity. As stated in chapter 1, clinical hypertension begins at that level where clinical intervention is beneficial to the individual patient. In contrast, the view of blood pressure from the public health perspective would imply a need to reduce the average blood pressure of the whole population and not just those individuals with abnormally increased blood pressures.

Systolic and diastolic blood pressures

In people older than 45 years, the risks of stroke and coronary heart disease are related more closely to systolic blood pressure, even after adjustment for underlying diastolic blood pressure. Isolated systolic hypertension thus becomes more common with increasing age and may be the result of thickening of the brachial artery, which would reflect arterial damage. Even in the presence of a normal or low diastolic blood pressure, systolic hypertension is an accurate predictor of cardiovascular risk.

It remains possible that diastolic pressure may be more important than systolic pressure in younger adults, although not much data on this point exist. In addition, diastolic pressure may exert its harmful effects only above a certain threshold of around 110 mm Hg. A blood pressure of 200/100 mm Hg thus may be less harmful than a blood pressure of 180/120 mm Hg.

The relative risks of stroke according to categories of baseline blood pressure in 6545 people who participated in the Copenhagen City Heart Study show that the highest risk is

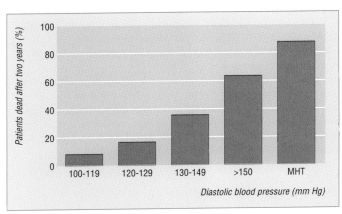

Severe hypertension in untreated patients. MHT=malignant hypertension

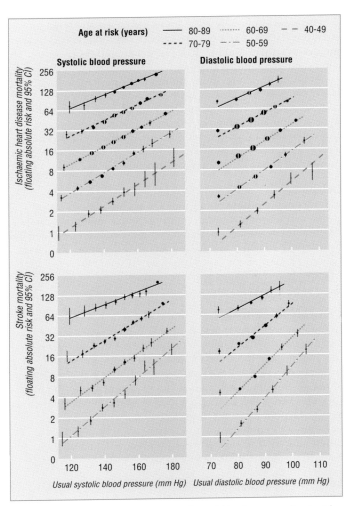

Mortality from coronary heart disease and usual blood pressure (top) and mortality from stroke and usual blood pressure (bottom)

present in people with isolated systolic hypertension and systolic diastolic hypertension, while isolated diastolic hypertension seems to carry a lower risk. Isolated diastolic hypertension is relatively uncommon and is usually seen in younger people, in whom the number of cardiovascular events is small. The significance of isolated diastolic hypertension in the long term remains uncertain.

High systolic and diastolic blood pressures are treatable cardiovascular risk factors. Good detection, treatment, and control result in a substantial reduction in the numbers of heart attacks and strokes.

Many patients are unaware that they have hypertension until they develop its complications: stroke, heart disease, peripheral vascular disease, renal failure, and retinopathy. The effective detection and treatment of hypertension is vital to reduce the incidence of cardiovascular disease. Special efforts have to be made to improve the efficiency of healthcare delivery.

Stroke

Stroke is one of the most devastating consequences of hypertension and results in premature death or considerable disability. About 80% of strokes in patients with hypertension are ischaemic, being caused by an intra-arterial thrombosis or embolisation from the heart or carotid arteries. The remaining 20% of cases are the result of various haemorrhagic causes. In the United Kingdom, about 40% of all strokes are attributable to systolic blood pressures ≥140 mm Hg. After adjustment for age, men aged 40–59 years with systolic blood pressures of 160–180 mm Hg are at about a fourfold higher risk of stroke during the next eight years than men with systolic blood pressures of 140–159 mm Hg.

Hypertension also is associated with an increased risk of atrial fibrillation. The presence of both conditions is additive to the risk of stroke. The incidence of stroke in patients with both conditions is 8% per year.

Abundant evidence from clinical trials shows that lowering blood pressure prevents all kinds of stroke. It has been commented that stroke should no longer occur as a result of hypertension and that when it does, it is a marker for poor control of blood pressure and inferior healthcare provision. Recent evidence suggests that the β blockers are less effective at preventing stroke than other antihypertensive agents.

Dementia

Elderly people with hypertension are at risk of all forms of stroke and frequently sustain multiple small, asymptomatic cerebral infarcts that may lead to progressive loss of intellectual or cognitive function and dementia. An association also exists between hypertension and Alzheimer's disease. Evidence as to whether lowering blood pressure leads to a reduction of dementia or loss of cognitive function is conflicting.

Coronary heart disease

In patients with hypertension, fatal coronary heart disease was more common than fatal stroke, but recent trends suggest a reversal of these frequencies. Adequate treatment of hypertension reduces the risk of heart attack by about 20%, although this figure is based on blood pressure lowering by thiazides and β blockers rather than newer antihypertensive agents. Hypertension may lead to coronary heart disease because of its contribution to the formation of coronary atheromas, with an interaction with other risk factors such as hyperlipidaemia and diabetes mellitus.

Left ventricular hypertrophy

Left ventricular hypertrophy occurs as a result of increased afterload on the heart, caused by more peripheral

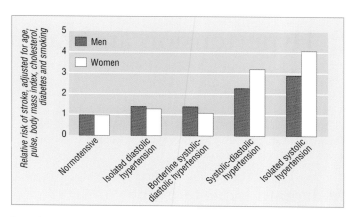

Copenhagen city heart study—relative risk of stroke with normotension, isolated diastolic hypertension, isolated systolic hypertension, and systolic-diastolic hypertension, and isolated systolic hypertension

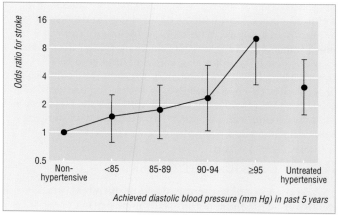

Blood pressure control and odds ratio for stroke in study of 267 cases and 534 controls

Stroke versus heart attack in long-term outcome trials

Trial	Mean age (years)	Event	
		Stroke	Heart attack
CAPPP	53	340	327
HOT	61	294	209
INSIGHT	67	141	138
LIFE	67	541	386
NICS	70	20	4
NORDIL	60	355	340
SHEP	72	269	165
STONE	67	52	4
STOP	76	82	53
Syst-China	67	104	16
Syst-Eur	70	124	78
STOP-2	76	452	293

CAPPP = Captopril Prevention Project; HOT = Hypertension Optimal Treatment; INSIGHT = International Nifedipine GITS Study: Intervention as a Goal in Hypertension Treatment; LIFE = Losartan Intervention For Endpoint Reduction; NICS = National Intervention Cooperative Study; NORDIL = Nordic Diltiazem; SHEP = Systolic Hypertension in the Elderly Program; STONE = Shanghai Trial of Hypertension in the Elderly; STOP-Hypertension = Swedish Trial in Old Patients with Hypertension; Syst-China = Systolic Hypertension in the Elderly: Chinese trial; Syst-Eur = Systolic Hypertension in Europe.

vascular resistance. Subsequently, the increased muscle mass outstrips its blood supply and this, coupled with the decreased coronary vascular reserve, can result in myocardial ischaemia—even in patients with normal coronary arteries. Evidence also shows that a high intake of salt and increased levels of angiotensin II in the plasma increase the chances of developing left ventricular hypertrophy. The angiotensin blocking drugs reduce left ventricular hypertrophy more than other classes of drug. The prevalence of left ventricular hypertrophy is similar in patients with isolated systolic hypertension and systolic-diastolic hypertension.

Left ventricular hypertrophy secondary to hypertension is a major risk factor for myocardial infarction, stroke, sudden death, and congestive cardiac failure. This increased risk is in addition to that imposed by hypertension itself. In addition, patients with hypertension and left ventricular hypertrophy are at increased risk of cardiac arrhythmias (atrial fibrillation and ventricular arrhythmias) and atherosclerotic vascular disease (coronary and peripheral artery disease). When left ventricular hypertrophy is accompanied by repolarisation abnormalities (also called "strain" pattern), morbidity and mortality are even higher.

Heart failure

In many epidemiological studies, such as the Framingham Heart Study, hypertension is the principal cause of heart failure. People with blood pressure >160/95 mm Hg have a sixfold higher incidence of heart failure than those with pressures <140/90 mm Hg. Hypertension as a cause of heart failure, however, is confounded by the underlying predisposition to coronary artery disease. Most cases of heart failure are the result of left ventricular systolic dysfunction that results from damage to the ventricle after myocardial infarction.

The presence of left ventricular hypertrophy on an electrocardiogram itself significantly increases the risk of heart failure. The development of atrial fibrillation can precipitate heart failure, especially if left ventricular hypertrophy and diastolic dysfunction are present. The presence of gross left ventricular hypertrophy can result in impaired ventricular compliance and relaxation, which leads to diastolic heart failure or "heart failure with normal systolic function."

Finally, hypertension in association with renal artery stenosis but with no intrinsic myocardial disease can cause "flash" pulmonary oedema that is related to high levels of plasma renin and angiotensin. This can be corrected by treatment of the renal artery stenosis.

Over many years, heart failure in association with untreated hypertension may lead slowly to a decrease in blood pressure as the left ventricular function progressively worsens. Patients whose hypertension mysteriously has normalised may have a bad outlook, as this normalisation is the result of a silent or clinically overt myocardial infarction or the development of left ventricular systolic dysfunction.

Large vessel arterial disease

Hypertension contributes to atheromatous vascular disease in all vascular beds. Peripheral artery disease manifested by intermittent claudication is about three times more common in patients with hypertension. Such patients also may have renal artery stenosis, which may contribute to their hypertension. Disease in the aorta coupled with hypertension may result in the development of abdominal aortic aneurysms. High pulsatile wave stress and atheromatous disease can lead to dissection of aortic aneurysms, which carries a high short term mortality. Extracranial carotid artery disease also is more common in people with hypertension.

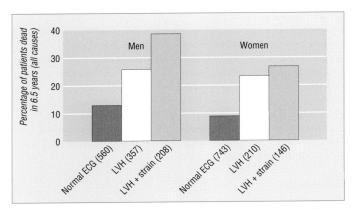

Mortality in patients with left ventricular hypertrophy with repolarisation abnormalities (strain) on echocardiograms in the blood pressure clinic at Glasgow. (ECG = echocardiogram, LVH = left ventricular hypertrophy)

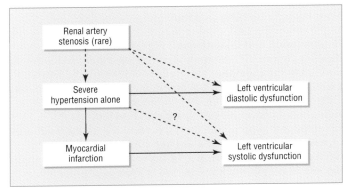

Mechanisms of heart failure in hypertension

Blood pressure and risk of intermittent claudication

Risk factor	Relative risk (95% CI) of intermittent claudication
Systolic blood pressure ≥160 mm Hg	3.4 (2.3 to 6.9)
Diastolic blood pressure ≥90 mm Hg	3.2 (1.9 to 11.6)
Smoking ≥15 cigarettes per day	8.8 (3.0 to 25.6)

Adapted from Hughson M. *BMJ* 1978;1:1379–81

Prevalence of abdominal aortic aneurysm in patients with hypertension

Study	Prevalence (%)
Scriffen, 1995	11.9
Vardulaki, 2000	4.8
Spittel, 1997	6.5
Lindholt, 1997	17.8
Williams, 1996:	
Men	5.2
Women	0.1
Grimshaw, 1994	7.7%

Adapted from Makin AJ. *J Human Hypertens* 2001;15:447–54

Renal disease

Renal dysfunction commonly is associated with hypertension, although some controversy exists as to whether mild to moderate essential hypertension leads to renal failure. This is because it remains unclear whether people with hypertension who develop progressive renal failure may have had undiagnosed primary renal disease in the first place. Malignant hypertension often leads to progressive renal failure. Almost all primary renal diseases cause an increase in blood pressure, which is mediated by high levels of renin and angiotensin, as well as sodium and water retention.

Retinopathy

Hypertension leads to vascular changes in the eye, which is referred to as hypertensive retinopathy. These changes were classified by Keith, Wagener, and Barker into four grades that correlate with prognosis. The most severe hypertension—that is, malignant hypertension—is defined clinically as increased blood pressure in association with bilateral retinal flame shaped haemorrhages and cotton wool spots or hard exudates, or both, with or without papilloedema. If untreated, 88% of patients with malignant hypertension die within two years—mainly from heart failure, renal failure, or stroke.

Hypertension and anaesthesia

Patients with severe hypertension are at increased risk of events during the intraoperative and postoperative periods, with a high incidence of myocardial infarction and arrhythmias. Some evidence shows that β blockers given immediately before anaesthesia reduce this risk. If patients have only mild asymptomatic hypertension and are otherwise generally fit with no evidence of target organ damage (for example, no electrocardiographic evidence of left ventricular hypertrophy), the risk in the perioperative period is likely to be minimal. Thus, many non-urgent surgical operations in such patients are postponed unnecessarily.

Multiple risk factors

High blood pressure should not be viewed as a risk factor in isolation. Instead, patients with hypertension very often have many additional risk factors, including hyperlipidaemia, diabetes mellitus, and impaired glucose tolerance. Patients with hypertension who smoke cigarettes are at particularly high risk.

  The treatment of people with hypertension should not focus solely on blood pressure but must also assess total risk for cardiovascular disease and use multifactorial interventions to reduce their risk in a "holistic" approach. The treatment of blood pressure alone in the presence of other risk factors may be relatively ineffective at preventing stroke and myocardial infarction. Coexistent signs of cardiovascular end organ damage also confer a high degree of cardiovascular risk on a patient. For example, left ventricular hypertrophy, previous heart attack, and stroke are all major contributors to premature death.

How do we assess risk of cardiovascular disease?

The risk of cardiovascular disease can be assessed in many different ways. These include "gut feeling" (commonly practised in the clinic but not very scientific), various complex algorithms (used more as research tools than for everyday clinical use), and simple colour charts that are based on established risk scores.

  The British Hypertension Society's guidelines recommend the use of a total cardiovascular disease risk chart that was initially issued by the Joint British Societies (the British Cardiac Society, British Hyperlipidaemia Association, British

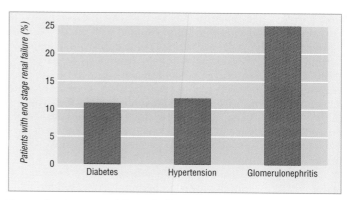

Causes of end stage renal disease in Europe

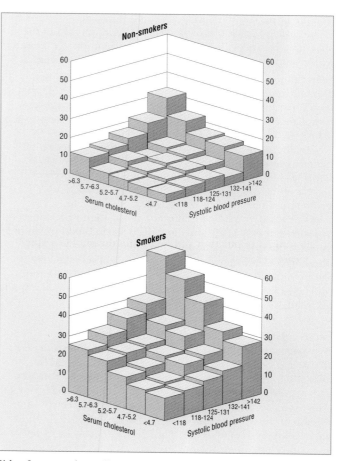

Risks of coronary heart disease and stroke in relation to smoking status, serum cholesterol levels, and systolic blood pressure mortality per 10 000 person years in MRFIT screenees

Hypertension Society, and endorsed by the British Diabetic Association) to estimate the risk of cardiovascular disease at 10 years. These risk charts quantify three levels of risk at 10 years, which are represented by three colour bands on the accompanying colour chart.

The Joint British Societies cardiovascular risk prediction charts (see appendix) are based on the long term follow up of people in the town of Framingham, Massachusetts. Whether the charts are applicable to populations of non-European origin in whom patterns of cardiovascular disease are different is uncertain. In people of African and Far Eastern origin, strokes outnumber heart attacks, and these important differences in cardiovascular disease may not be explained by the risk factors measured in the Framingham study. These charts, however, do at least take into account multiple risk factors and can be used to explain risk status to patients and their doctors. They can be used as a rough guide in patients of non-European origin.

Risk factor assessment in the clinic
Smoking and hyperlipidaemia
The two most important independent risk factors that need to be taken into consideration are smoking and hyperlipidaemia. In combination with hypertension, these two risk factors have a synergistic effect. Thus, a patient with mild hypertension who does not smoke and has a normal ratio of serum total cholesterol to high density lipoprotein cholesterol has a much lower risk of cardiovascular disease than a patient with mild hypertension who also smokes and has an increased serum cholesterol/high density lipoprotein cholesterol ratio.

Another factor to take into consideration when deciding about whether to treat hypertension is the patient's age. Although the relative risk of mortality from cardiovascular disease in a young man with mild hypertension is increased, the absolute risk of him sustaining a stroke or myocardial infarction within the next 10 years may be low. For an elderly patient with the same degree of hypertension, however, the absolute risk of stroke or heart attack is much higher, as the prevalence of these conditions increases with age. In addition, up to the age of about 50 years, women have a lower risk of cardiovascular disease than men.

Public health approach
In contrast to the strategy of assessing a patient's personal risk when making the decision to start treatment, the public health approach to hypertension means that we should consider community risk on the basis of evidence that the risk of cardiovascular disease increases with blood pressures even within the normotensive range. Most heart attacks and strokes occur in people with blood pressures that are around average for the general population and below the threshold at which drug treatment would be reasonable. It seems appropriate to try to reduce the blood pressure of the community as a whole. A shift in the entire bell shaped distribution curve of blood pressure by 5 mm Hg to the left would be expected to produce about a 40% reduction in the incidence of stroke and a 20–25% reduction of coronary heart disease.

Two strategies thus exist for prevention of cardiovascular disease. Patient care is the strategy of treating people with a high risk. In contrast, the public health strategy can be achieved only by public education and manipulation of the nation's habits—sometimes by means of legislation on food labelling. This population based approach aims to produce radical alterations in the national diet, with lower intakes of salt and animal fat and higher intakes of fruit and vegetables. More people should be encouraged to take more exercise and moderate their alcohol consumption, and, of course, benefits can be gained from a reduction of passive and active smoking.

Problems inherent in the total cardiovascular risk chart recommended by the British Hypertension Society

- The chart predicts absolute risk at 10 years, which results in a tendency to undertreat young people at high relative risk and overtreat older people at lower relative risk
  —For example, a woman aged 32 years—even with diabetes, a current smoking history, a total cholesterol:high density lipoprotein cholesterol ratio of 8, and a systolic blood pressure of 170 mm Hg—does not reach the 30% threshold of risk of cardiovascular disease at 10 years
  —Most elderly men would have qualified for intervention simply on account of their age and sex
- Until 2005, the colour charts published in the *British National Formulary* showed the risk of coronary heart disease (CHD) not the total risk of cardiovascular disease
  —This meant the risk of stroke was ignored
  —This serious error has now been corrected to quantitate total cardiovascular disease (CVD) risk

---

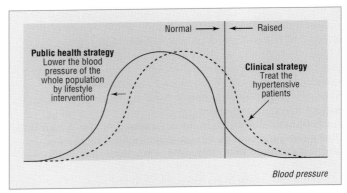

Public health and clinical reductions in blood pressure

The figure showing severe hypertension in untreated patients uses data taken from Leishman AWD. *BMJ* 1959;1:1361–3. The figures showing mortality from coronary heart disease and usual blood pressure and mortality from stroke and usual blood pressure are adapted from the Prospective Studies Collaboration. *Lancet* 2002;360:1903–13. The figure of relative risk of stroke with normotension, isolated diastolic hypertension, isolated systolic hypertension, and systolic-diastolic hypertension, and isolated systolic hypertension uses data from the Copenhagen city heart study and adapted from Nielsen N, et al. *Am J Hypertens* 1997;10:634–9. The figure of blood pressure and odds ratio for stroke is adapted from Du X, et al. *BMJ* 1997;314:272. The figure showing mortality in patients with left ventricular hypertrophy with repolarisation abnormalities on echocardiograms is adapted from Dunn FG, et al. *J Hypertens* 1990;8:775–82. The figure showing causes of end stage renal disease in Europe is adapted from United States renal data system 1991. *Nephrol Dialysis Transplant* 1995;10:1–25. The figure showing risks of coronary heart disease in relation to smoking status, serum cholesterol levels, and systolic blood pressure in the MRFIT study is adapted from Stamler J, et al. *JAMA* 1986;256:2823–8

11

3 Pathophysiology of hypertension

G Y H Lip, D G Beevers

A few patients (2–5%) have an underlying renal or adrenal disease as the cause for their increased blood pressure. In the remaining patients, no cause is found, and such cases are referred to as having "essential hypertension." This is clearly illogical, as all diseases have a cause or causes. A wide variety of pathophysiological mechanisms are involved in the maintenance of blood pressure, and their derangement thus may result in the development of essential hypertension.

Balance between cardiac output and peripheral resistance

Blood pressure is normally dependent on the balance between cardiac output and peripheral resistance. Most patients with essential hypertension have increased peripheral vascular resistance and a normal cardiac output. The cardiac output may be increased in the early stages of essential hypertension, so that the peripheral resistance gradually increases in order to maintain normal tissue perfusion and cardiac output returns to normal. In the end stages of hypertension, left ventricular damage becomes so severe that cardiac output decreases, so that blood pressure is maintained solely by increased peripheral vascular resistance. At the final stage, the cardiac output may be so impaired that blood pressure then decreases, rendering the patient frankly hypotensive.

Peripheral resistance is not determined by the large arteries or the capillaries but by the small arterioles. The walls of these arterioles contain smooth muscle cells. Extrinsic influences result in contraction of these smooth muscle cells, probably mediated ultimately by a rise in intracellular levels of calcium. Drugs that block the calcium channels thus have a vasodilatory effect that decreases blood pressure. In people with chronic hypertension, the prolonged constriction of smooth muscle results in structural changes to the arterioles, with thickening of the walls and a further increase in arterial blood pressure.

Renin-angiotensin-aldosterone system

The renin-angiotensin-aldosterone system is one of the major hormonal systems that influence blood pressure. Two of the main drug classes for the treatment of hypertension—the angiotensin converting enzyme inhibitors and the angiotensin receptor blockers—specifically target this system. The hormone aldosterone also can be antagonised by drugs such as spironolactone, but despite beneficial effects in patients with heart failure, little evidence shows a benefit when they are used alone in patients with essential hypertension.

Renin is secreted from the juxtaglomerular apparatus of the kidney in response to glomerular underperfusion, reduced intake of salt, or stimulation from the sympathetic nervous system. Renin results in the conversion of renin substrate (angiotensinogen) to angiotensin I, which is a physiologically inactive substance. A key enzyme, angiotensin converting enzyme (ACE), results in the conversion of angiotensin I to angiotensin II.

Angiotensin II is a potent vasoconstrictor that leads to an increase in blood pressure. Angiotensin II may also cause some of the manifestations of hypertensive target organ damage,

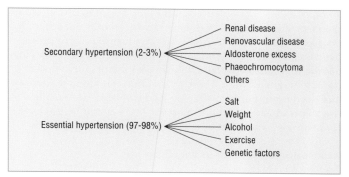

Aetiology of hypertension

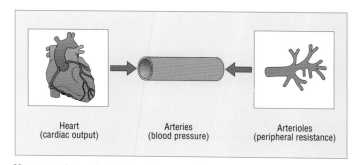

Heart, arteries, and arterioles in hypertension

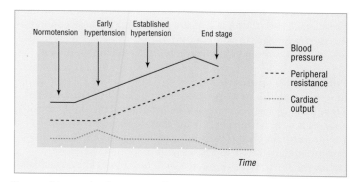

Proposed interaction between cardiac output and peripheral vascular resistance in pathogenesis of essential hypertension

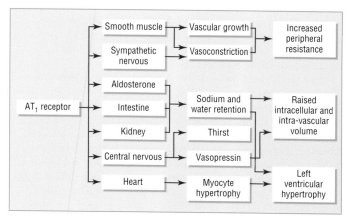

Actions of angiotensin II mediated by the angiotensin I (AT₁) receptor

such as left ventricular hypertrophy and atherosclerotic vascular disease. Hypertension that results directly from excess renin and aldosterone is seen in patients with renin secreting tumours and in some cases of renal artery stenosis.

Angiotensin II also stimulates release of aldosterone from the zona glomerulosa of the adrenal gland. Aldosterone causes fluid and sodium retention, and this results in a further increase in blood pressure.

The renin-angiotensin system, however, is not thought to be responsible directly for the increase in blood pressure in patients with essential hypertension. Many patients with hypertension have low levels of circulating endocrine renin and angiotensin II, and, in these patients, the drugs that block the renin-angiotensin-aldosterone system tend to be less effective.

Evidence shows that non-circulating levels of "local" or "tissue" angiotensin contribute to control of blood pressure; these hormones are classified as epicrine or paracrine rather than endocrine. Examples are the local renin systems in the kidney and arterial tree, which have important roles in the regulation of regional blood flow. Although some drugs have particular affinity for angiotensin converting enzyme in tissue, differences in affinity have not translated to marked differences in clinical outcomes.

Volume mediated hypertension

Patients with hypertension and low levels of renin and angiotensin tend to be older and more often of African origin. In these patients, volume overload may cause hypertension. Volume mediated hypertension is also seen in patients with primary excess of aldosterone (for example, Conn's syndrome) and type 2 diabetes.

In most other patients, plasma levels of renin, angiotensin and aldosterone are not increased, and circulating blood volume, total body water, and total exchangeable sodium are normal. In these people, hypertension may be related to an interplay between blood volume and renin-angiotensin mediated vasoconstriction.

Autonomic nervous system

The second main neurohumeral system that influences blood pressure is the sympathetic nervous system and the corresponding plasma catecholamines. The autonomic nervous system thus has an important role in maintaining a "normal" blood pressure, including the physiological responses to changes in posture, as well as physical and emotional activity.

Stimulation of the sympathetic nervous system can cause arteriolar constriction and arteriolar dilatation. After stress and physical exercise, such changes mediate short term changes in blood pressure.

Only limited evidence suggests that the catecholamines (adrenaline and noradrenaline) have a clear role in essential hypertension. Exceptions are the rare catecholamine secreting tumours, such as phaeochromocytoma, which can cause severe secondary hypertension.

Nevertheless, the effects of the sympathetic nervous system are important, as drugs that act on this system decrease blood pressure. The importance of activation of the sympathetic system in heart failure as a result of systolic dysfunction and in progression of and mortality from renal insufficiency is well established. For example, the role of β blockers in patients with chronic heart failure is well established to improve mortality and morbidity.

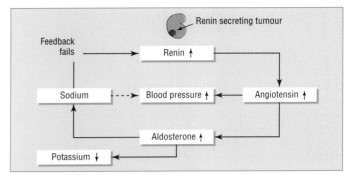

Hypertension as a result of isolated excess of renin as seen with renin secreting tumours, renal artery stenosis, and some primary renal diseases

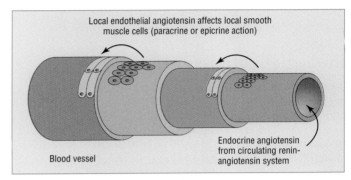

Local versus systematic renin-angiotensin systems

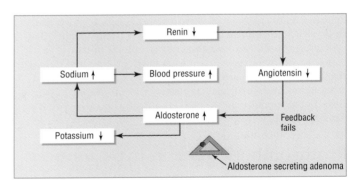

Hypertension caused by an isolated excess of aldosterone

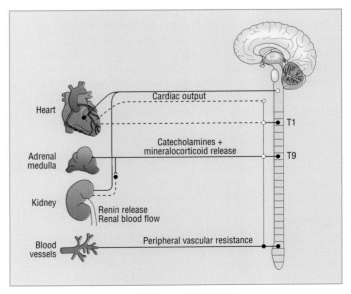

Autonomic nervous system and its control of blood pressure

Insulin sensitivity and metabolic syndrome

In 1988, Reaven highlighted the frequent clustering of multiple risk factors, particularly, increased blood pressure, dyslipidaemia, abnormal glucose regulation, and obesity. This cluster of cardiovascular risk factors was termed "syndrome X," "insulin resistance syndrome," "metabolic syndrome," or sometimes "Reaven's syndrome."

Metabolic syndrome is common in high risk populations, and an alarming prevalence of 24% has been documented in the American population. Mortality from cardiovascular and peripheral vascular disease is higher in people with metabolic syndrome than in those without. Metabolic syndrome particularly is prevalent in people of South Asian (Indian, Pakistani, and Bangladeshi) and African-Caribbean origin, who have high morbidity and mortality from vascular disease.

Endothelial function

Interest in the role of the endothelium in vascular disease has been extensive, and the traditional belief that the endothelium is an inert interface between blood and the vessel wall is no longer held. The endothelium produces an extensive range of substances that influence blood flow and, in turn, is affected by changes in the blood and the pressure of blood flow. For example, local nitric oxide and endothelin, which are secreted by the endothelium, are the major regulators of vascular tone and blood pressure.

In patients with essential hypertension, the balance between the vasodilators and the vasoconstrictors is upset, which leads to changes in the endothelium and sets up a "vicious cycle" that contributes to the maintenance of high blood pressure. In patients with hypertension, endothelial activation and damage also lead to changes in vascular tone, vascular reactivity, and coagulation and fibrinolytic pathways. Alterations in endothelial function are a reliable indicator of target organ damage and atherosclerotic disease, as well as prognosis.

Prothrombotic state in hypertension

Although patients with high blood pressure have high intra-arterial pressures, their vessels tend more often to thrombose than burst. Cerebral infarction is therefore much more common than cerebral haemorrhage.

Nearly 150 years ago, Virchow postulated a triad of abnormalities that predispose to thrombus formation (thrombogenesis). These are abnormalities in blood flow, blood constituents, and the vessel wall. These are referred to as "Virchow's triad." Evidence suggests that hypertension fulfils the prerequisites of Virchow's triad for thrombogenesis, which leads to a prothrombotic or hypercoagulable state. For example, hypertension leads to changes in platelets, the endothelium, and the coagulation-fibrinolytic pathways that promote the induction and maintenance of this prothrombotic state. These changes can be reversed, to a certain extent, by the treatment of hypertension, although different antihypertensive agents may have variable effects in reversing these changes.

Angiogenesis

Angiogenesis is increasingly recognised as an important aspect of the pathophysiology of cardiovascular disease and has an impact on thrombogenesis and atherogenesis. The process of thrombogenesis is related intimately to atherogenesis. A common feature is loss of integrity of the endothelial cells. Certainly, endothelial damage or dysfunction is crucial in the

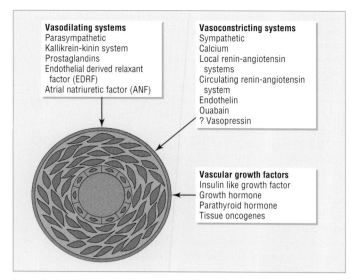

Control of peripheral arteriolar resistance

Thrombotic paradox of hypertension (Birmingham Paradox)

Although the blood vessels in patients with hypertension are exposed to increased internal pressure, the main complications of hypertension—namely heart attack and stroke—are thrombotic rather than haemorrhagic in origin

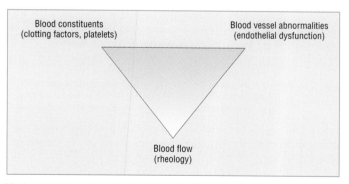

Virchow's triad and prothrombotic state in hypertension

Essential hypertension is characterised by an impaired capacity for vascular growth, as well as structural alterations of microvascular beds

formation of atherosclerosis (atherogenesis). Angiogenesis is another pathophysiological process that is also evident in atherosclerotic vascular disease: vasa vasorum in the adventitia and media are at a higher density in atherosclerotic tissue and often greater neovascularisation is seen, which leads to stenoses or collateral growth to bypass obstructions, or both.

Salt sensitivity

The precise mechanism of salt induced increases in blood pressure—a phenomenon known as "salt sensitivity"—is understood incompletely. Indeed, the effect of salt in essential hypertension is not predicted by the level of salt intake, but perhaps by the salt sensitivity. Recent evidence suggests that salt sensitivity is an independent risk factor for hypertensive target organ damage and cardiovascular morbidity and mortality. Certainly, restriction of salt intake reduces blood pressure and increases sensitivity to antihypertensive drugs during treatment of hypertension, but wide differences in salt sensitivity are seen when individuals are compared.

Natriuretic peptides

Atrial natriuretic peptide (ANP) is a hormone secreted from the atria of the heart in response to increased blood volume. Increased levels of atrial natriuretic peptide result in an increase in excretion of sodium (and fluid) from the kidney. A defect in this system theoretically may cause fluid retention and hypertension.

Brain natriuretic peptide (BNP) is a hormone produced by the left ventricle and has gained much interest as a marker for the presence of left ventricular systolic dysfunction. Brain natriuretic peptide has been promoted as a "blood test" with a high negative predictive value for heart failure secondary to systolic dysfunction. Increased levels of brain natriuretic peptide have been related to left ventricular hypertrophy and reduced ventricular compliance (so called "diastolic dysfunction").

Genes and hypertension

Each person's variance in blood pressure is under an important degree of genetic control, but quantitative estimates range from 35% to 70%. About 50% of patients with hypertension have a family history of high blood pressure or premature death from cardiac problems in first degree relatives. People with normal blood pressure but a strong family history of hypertension are at a greater risk than those with no such history. The precise identification of "genes that cause hypertension" has not been clear, however, because of the multifactorial nature of the disease and the presence of many major pathogenetic pathways. Indeed, major genes that definitely cause essential hypertension have yet to be discovered, although more than 20 published genomewide screens are available for genes that control blood pressure. Some autosomal dominant genetically inherited forms of hypertension exist, but they are very rare.

Intrauterine growth and hypertension

The "Barker hypothesis" postulates that hypertension and related risk factors for cardiovascular disease—including central obesity, hyperlipidaemia, glucose intolerance, and type 2 diabetes—can originate through impaired growth and development during fetal life. The hypothesis suggests that hypertension and related risk factors for cardiovascular disease may be the consequences of "programming," whereby a stimulus or insult at a specific, critical, sensitive period of early

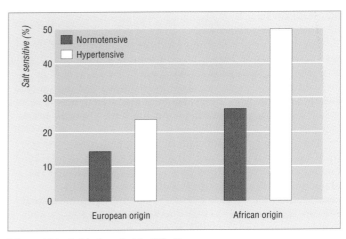

Salt sensitivity in black and white US citizens

Salt sensitivity is likely to be distributed in a Gaussian or "normal" distribution rather than a dichotomous division of patients who are salt sensitive or salt resistant

---

Examples of specific genetic mutations that cause hypertension

- **Liddle's syndrome**—a disorder associated with hypertension, low plasma levels of renin and aldosterone, and hypokalaemia: all of which respond to amiloride, an inhibitor of the distal renal epithelial sodium channel
- **Glucocorticoid remediable aldosterone**—a disorder that mimics Conn's syndrome, in which a chimeric gene is formed from portions of the 11β-hydroxylase gene and the aldosterone synthase gene. This defect results in hyperaldosteronism, which is responsive to dexamethasone and has a high incidence of stroke
- **Congenital adrenal hyperplasia due to 11β-hydroxylase deficiency**—a disorder that has been associated with 10 different mutations of the CYP11B1 gene
- **Syndrome of apparent mineralocorticoid excess**—this disorder arises from mutations in the gene that encodes the kidney enzyme 11α-hydroxysteroid dehydrogenase. The defective enzyme allows normal circulating levels of cortisol (which are much higher than those of aldosterone) to activate the mineralocorticoid receptors
- **Congenital adrenal hyperplasia due to 17α-hydroxylase deficiency**—a disorder with hyporeninaemia hypoaldosteronism, absent secondary sexual characteristics, and hypokalaemia
- **Gordon's syndrome** (pseudo-hypoaldosteronism)—familial hypertension with hyperkalaemia, which possibly is related to the long arm of chromosome 17
- Sporadic case reports of familial inheritance of phaeochromocytoma (multiple endocrine neoplasia (MEN-2) syndrome), Cushing's syndrome, Conn's syndrome, and renal artery stenosis as a result of fibromuscular dysplasia

Other associations
- Angiotensinogen gene may be related to hypertension
- Angiotensin converting enzyme gene may be related to left ventricular hypertrophy or hypertensive nephropathy
- α-Adducin gene may be related to salt sensitive hypertension
- Autosomal dominant polycystic kidney disease (PKD-1 and PKD-2)—a primary renal disease that frequently causes hypertension

life results in long term changes in specific aspects of physiology and metabolism.

Low birth weight and other indices of abnormal growth in utero are related to higher blood pressure, glucose intolerance, and other risk factors for cardiovascular disease, as well as increased risk of cardiovascular disease events and mortality in later life. People who were small and thin at birth are therefore at particularly high risk of hypertension if they become obese in adult life.

The Barker hypothesis cannot fully explain observations from many cross population studies of the effects of migration and acculturation on blood pressure and cardiovascular risk. Many other influencing confounding factors are still unaccounted for, including social class at birth and maternal risk factors for cardiovascular disease during pregnancy, such as maternal blood pressure. For example, high-normal maternal blood pressure during pregnancy is associated with low normal birth weight and plausibly with hypertension in later life through the genes and environment shared by a mother and her offspring.

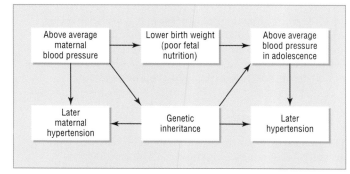

Possible mechanisms to explain why low birth weight babies are more likely to develop hypertension in later life

The figure of the autonomic nervous system and its control of blood pressure is adapted from Swales J, et al. *Clinical atlas of hypertension*. London and New York: Gower Medical Publishing, 1991. The figure of control of peripheral arteriolar resistance is adapted from Beevers DG, MacGregor GA. *Hypertension in practice*. London: Martin Dunitz, 1999. The figure of salt sensitivity in black and white US citizens is adapted from Sullivan JM, et al. *Am J Med Sci* 1998;295:370–7

4 Measurement of blood pressure

Eoin O'Brien

Part I: Aspects of measurement of blood pressure common to technique and patient

Technique

Selection of an accurate device

An accurate device is fundamental to all measurements of blood pressure. If the device is inaccurate, attention to the detail of measurement methods is of little relevance. The accuracy of devices for measurement of blood pressure should not be judged on the sole basis of claims from manufacturers, which can be extravagant. Instead devices should be validated according to international protocols in peer reviewed journals.

> The website dableducational provides updated assessments of all devices used to measure blood pressure and indicates which have passed or failed independent validation (see example table below—for full details go to www.dableducational.org)

Sphygmomanometers for self-measurement of blood pressure—devices for the upper arm

Device	Mode of measurement	AAMI	BHS	ESH	Circumstance	Recommendation
A&D UA-631 (UA-779 Life Source)	Oscillometric			Pass	At rest, recruitment violations	Recommended
A&D UA-704	Oscillometric		A/A		Study details omitted	Questionable
A&D UA-767	Oscillometric	Pass	A/A		At rest; not high blood pressure	Recommended
A&D UA-767 Plus	Oscillometric		A/A		At rest; tables incomplete	Recommended
			A/A		At rest; recruitment violations	Questionable
			A/A		At rest; recruitment violations; simultaneous readings	Questionable
A&D UA-787	Oscillometric			Pass		Recommended
Microlife BP 3AC1-1	Oscillometric			Pass		Recommended
Microlife BP 3BTO-A	Oscillometric		A/A		Small recruitment violation	Recommended
		Pass	A/B		Normotensive pregnancy	Recommended
		Pass	B/B		Non-proteinuric high blood pressure	
		Pass	A/B		Pre-eclampsia	
Omron HEM-705IT	Oscillometric			Pass		Recommended
Omron M5-I	Oscillometric			Pass		Recommended
Omron MX3 Plus	Oscillometric			Pass	Recruitment ranges omitted; from plot, high range of diastolic blood pressure seems undersubscribed	Questionable
Rossmax	Oscillometric on inflation			Fail	At rest	Not recommended
Visomat OZ2	Oscillometric	Pass	C/B		At rest	Not recommended
Welch-Allyn transtelephonic home monitor	Oscillometric	Pass			Parkinson's disease	Questionable

AAMI = American Association of Medical Instrumentation; BHS = British Hypertension Society; ESH = European Society for Hypertension. Table adapted from dabl® Educational Trust.

Variability of blood pressure

No matter which measurement device is used, blood pressure is always a variable haemodynamic phenomenon. Modification of the factors that influence variability is not always possible, but we can minimise their effect. When optimum conditions are not possible, this should be noted with the reading.

White coat hypertension and the white coat effect

Anxiety increases blood pressure—often by as much as 30 mm Hg—when patients are frightened and extremely anxious, when it is often referred to as the white coat effect. This effect should be distinguished from white coat hypertension, in which a person with normal blood pressure has hypertension during measurement by doctors and nurses but blood pressure returns to normal away from the medical environment. White coat

Factors that influence blood pressure variability

- Circumstances of measurement
- Respiration
- Emotion
- Exercise
- Meals
- Tobacco
- Alcohol
- Temperature
- Bladder distension
- Pain
- Age
- Race
- Diurnal variation (blood pressure lowest during sleep)

hypertension is shown best by ambulatory blood pressure measurement (Part III).

These white coat phenomena are important because a decision to reduce blood pressure, and especially to administer drugs, never should be made on the basis of measurements taken in circumstances in which the white coat effect or white coat hypertension is likely to occur.

Optimum conditions for measurement

- Relaxed patient
- Comfortable temperature
- Quiet room—no telephones or noises

Posture

Posture affects blood pressure, with a general tendency for it to decrease when a person moves from the lying position to the sitting or standing positions. Some patients may have postural hypotension, especially those who are taking certain antihypertensive drugs and elderly people. When this is likely, blood pressure should also be measured when the patient is standing.

Arm support

If the arm in which blood pressure is being measured is unsupported—as tends to happen when the patient is sitting or standing—the patient is performing isometric exercise, which increases blood pressure by as much as 10%. The arm therefore must be supported during measurement of blood pressure, especially when the patient is in the standing position. This is achieved best in practice by the observer holding the patient's arm at the elbow.

Arm position

The forearm should be at the level of the heart—that is, the mid-sternum. Measurement in an arm lower than the level of the heart leads to an overestimation of systolic and diastolic pressures, while measurement in an arm above the level of the heart leads to underestimation. Such inaccuracy can be as much as 10 mm Hg, especially when the patient is in the sitting or standing position, when the arm is likely to be below heart level by the side. Arm position is important for self measurement of blood pressure with devices for wrist measurement. Many of these devices inherently are inaccurate, but measurement is even less accurate if the wrist is not held at the level of the heart during measurement.

Which arm?

Arterial disease can cause differences in blood pressure between arms, but because blood pressure varies from beat to beat, any differences may simply reflect blood pressure variability or measurement errors, or both. Bilateral measurement should be made at the first consultation; if differences >20 mm Hg for systolic or 10 mm Hg for diastolic blood pressure are present on consecutive readings, the patient should be referred to a cardiovascular centre for further evaluation with simultaneous bilateral measurement and for the exclusion of arterial disease.

Cuff and bladder

The cuff is an inelastic cloth that encircles the arm and encloses an inflatable rubber bladder. The cuff is secured around the arm most often by means of Velcro on the adjoining surfaces of the cuff, occasionally by wrapping a tapering end into the encircling cuff, and rarely by hooks. Velcro surfaces must be effective; when they lose their grip, the

White coat phenomena

White coat effect

- Also known as: fight and flight phenomenon, alarm reaction, defence reaction
- Occurs in medical environment—for example, emergency department or surgery
- Occurs in people with normal blood pressure and hypertension
- Decreases with familiarisation

White coat hypertension

- Occurs in medical environment
- People with normal blood pressure become hypertensive. People with hypertension have higher blood pressures in a medical environment
- Tends to persist during repeated visits

Posture and position

- Measure blood pressure routinely with patient in sitting position
- Back should be supported
- Legs should be uncrossed
- Patient should be relaxed
- Measure after ten minutes of rest
- Measure after two minutes of standing if indicated

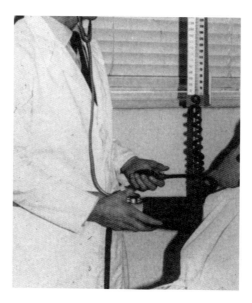

Arm support during blood pressure measurement

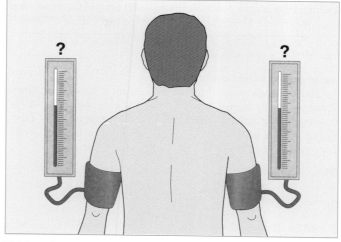

Which arm?

cuff should be discarded. The bladder should be removable from the cuff for washing.

Cuff hypertension

However sophisticated a blood pressure measuring device, if it is dependent on cuff occlusion of the arm (as most devices are), it will be prone to the inaccuracy of miscuffing. This occurs when a cuff contains a bladder that is too long or too short relative to the circumference of the patient's arm. Miscuffing is a serious source of error that leads inevitably to incorrect diagnosis in clinical practice and erroneous conclusions in research into hypertension. A further problem is that inflation of the cuff itself may result in a transient but substantial increase (up to 40 mm Hg) in the patient's blood pressure.

Solutions

Correction factors on the cuff to avoid measurement errors from an inappropriate bladder complicate blood pressure measurement and are not used often. Cuffs that contain a variety of bladders of varying dimensions are available (such as Tricuff, Pressure Group AB, Sweden), but they are expensive and can be difficult to apply because of stiffness of the cuff. A "universal" cuff adjustable for all arm dimensions has been proposed but not manufactured successfully yet.

A cuff that contains a bladder that measures 35 × 12 cm was used for a time on the basis that it would encircle most adult arms, but it introduced errors by overcuffing lean arms. Many national bodies now recommend a range of cuffs to cater for all eventualities, which presupposes that the user will measure the arm circumference and, having done so, will have access to an adequate range of cuffs. In practice, neither of these requirements is easily fulfilled.

Unfortunately, societies differ in their recommendations. The striking difference between the American and British recommendations is not so much the length of the bladders but the width: most European arms will comfortably accommodate a bladder with a width of 12 cm, but a bladder with a width of 16 cm is likely to encroach on the antecubital fossa—particularly if (as often happens in practice) the sleeve of the patient's shirt or blouse is rolled up.

The subject

Special management of blood pressure

Certain groups of people merit special consideration for the measurement of blood pressure because of age, body habitus, or disturbances of blood pressure related to haemodynamic alterations in the cardiovascular system.

Children

Measurement of blood pressure in children presents a number of difficulties. Variability of blood pressure is greater than in adults, and any one reading is less likely to represent the true blood pressure. Systolic pressure is more accurate and reproducible than diastolic pressure. A cuff with proper dimensions is essential for accurate measurement. The widest cuff practicable should be used.

Ideally, blood pressure should be measured after a few minutes of rest. Values obtained during sucking, crying, or eating will not be representative. As with adults, a child's blood pressure status should be decided only after it has been measured on a number of separate occasions.

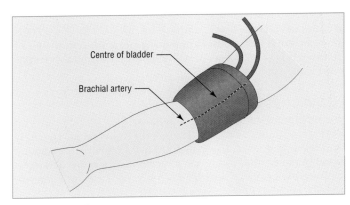

Placement of cuff

Mismatching of bladder and arm

Bladder too small (undercuffing)	Bladder too large (overcuffing)
• Overestimation of blood pressure	• Underestimation of blood pressure
• Range of error: —3/3 to 12/8 mm Hg —As much as 30 mm Hg in patients who are obese	• Range of error: —10–30 mm Hg

Undercuffing is more common than overcuffing

Cuffing solutions

- Correction factors on the cuff
- Cuffs containing a variety of bladders of varying dimensions
- A universal cuff for all arms
- A cuff suitable for most arms

Recommended bladder dimensions for adults

British Hypertension Society

Cuff type	For whom	Dimensions (cm)
Small	Lean adult arms and children	12 × 18
Standard	Most adult arms	12 × 26
Large	Arms of obese patients	12 × 40

American Heart Association

Cuff type	Arm circumference (cm)	Dimensions (cm)
Small adult	22−26	12 × 22
Adult	27−34	16 × 30
Large adult	35−44	16 × 36
Adult thigh	45−52	20 × 42

Recommended bladder dimensions for children aged 0–14 years

Cuff type	Dimensions (cm)
1	4 × 13
2	8 × 18
3	12 × 26

Korotkoff sounds are not audible reliably in any child younger than one year and in many children younger than five years, so Doppler ultrasound or oscillometry should be used

Body size is the most important determinant of blood pressure in childhood and adolescence. The US National High Blood Pressure Education Group on Hypertension Control in Children and Adolescents provides blood pressure ranges that relate to age and height.

Elderly people

In epidemiological and interventional studies, blood pressure predicts morbidity and mortality in elderly people as effectively as in the young. Elderly people have considerable variability in blood pressure, which can lead to a number of diurnal blood pressure patterns that are identified best with measurement of ambulatory blood pressure (see Part III).

Isolated systolic hypertension—This is the most common form of hypertension in elderly people.

Hypotension—Blood pressure in elderly people can vary greatly in those with autonomic failure, with periods of hypotension interspersed with hypertension on measurement of ambulatory blood pressure. As elderly people especially can be susceptible to the adverse effects of antihypertensive drugs, identification of postural hypotension particularly becomes important. Some elderly patients experience quite a marked decrease in blood pressure after eating, and this may be symptomatic. This again is diagnosed best by measurement of blood pressure when a patient is standing after a meal or with ambulatory blood pressure.

White coat hypertension—Elderly people are affected by the white coat phenomenon even more than young people.

Pseudohypertension—This term describes a large discrepancy between cuff and direct measurement of blood pressure in elderly patients. When conventional measurements seem to be out of proportion with the clinical findings, referral to a specialist cardiovascular centre for further investigation may be an appropriate option.

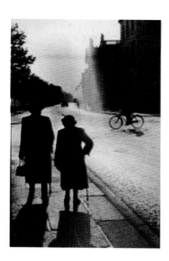

Blood pressure can vary considerably in elderly people. With permission from Nevill Johnson

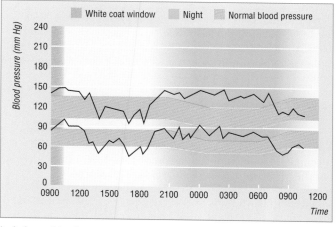

Ambulatory blood pressure measurement in a patient with hypotension. Plot and report generated by dabl ABPM— © dabl 2006 (www.dabl.ie)

Causes of hypotension in elderly patients

- Standing—postural hypotension
- Autonomic failure
- Drugs
- Meals—post-prandial hypotension
- Diabetes mellitus
- Parkinson's disease

Obese people

The association between obesity and hypertension has been confirmed in many epidemiological studies. Obesity may affect the accuracy of measurement of blood pressure in children, young and elderly people, and pregnant women. The relation of arm circumference to bladder dimensions is particularly important. If the bladder is too short, blood pressure will be overestimated—"cuff hypertension"—and if it is too long, blood pressure may be underestimated. The increasing prevalence of the metabolic syndrome, of which hypertension is a major component, means that accurate measurement of blood pressure increasingly becomes important.

Arrhythmias

Large variations in blood pressure from beat to beat make it difficult to obtain accurate measurements in patients with arrhythmias. In patients with arrhythmias such as atrial fibrillation, blood pressure varies depending on the preceding pulse interval. No generally accepted method of determining auscultatory endpoints in patients with arrhythmias exists.

International Diabetes Federation's consensus worldwide definition of metabolic syndrome (2005)

- Central obesity: waist >94 cm in men and >80 cm in women for Europids (figures available for other races)
- Two of the following:
  —Raised triglycerides: ≥1.7 mmol/l (or treatment)
  —Low levels of high density lipoprotein cholesterol: <1.04 mmol/l in men and <1.29 mmol/l in women (or treatment)
  —High blood pressure: ≥130/85 mm Hg (or treatment)
  —Fasting hyperglycaemia: glucose ≥5.6 mmol/l or previous diagnosis of diabetes or impaired glucose tolerance

Devices for measuring blood pressure vary greatly in their ability to accurately record blood pressure in patients with arrhythmias. Measurements of blood pressure at best will constitute a rough estimate in those with atrial fibrillation, particularly when the ventricular rhythm is rapid or highly irregular, or both. The rate of deflation should be no faster than 2 mm Hg per heartbeat, and repeated measurements may be needed to overcome variability from beat to beat.

Two potential sources of error exist when patients have bradyarrhythmia. If the rhythm is irregular, the same problems as with atrial fibrillation will apply. When the heart rate is extremely slow—for example 40 beats per minute—it is important that the rate of deflation used is less than for people with normal heart rates, as too rapid deflation will lead to underestimation of systolic blood pressure and overestimation of diastolic blood pressure.

Pregnancy

Clinically relevant hypertension occurs in more than 10% of pregnant women in most populations. High blood pressure is a key factor in medical decision making in pregnancy. Disappearance of sounds (fifth phase) is the most accurate measurement of diastolic pressure, except when sounds persist to zero, in which case the fourth phase of muffling of sounds should be used.

Patients who take antihypertensive drugs

In patients who take antihypertensive drugs, the timing of measurement may have a substantial influence on the blood pressure. The time of taking antihypertensive drugs should be noted.

Blood pressure in patients who are exercising

Systolic blood pressure increases with increasing dynamic work as a result of increasing cardiac output, whereas diastolic pressure usually remains about the same or moderately lower. An exaggerated blood pressure response during exercise may predict development of future hypertension.

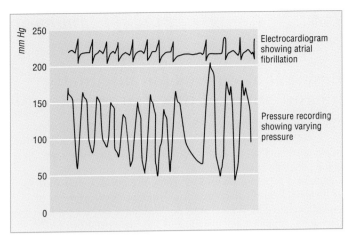

Atrial fibrillation

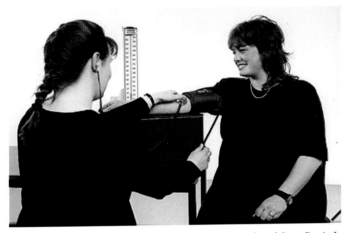

Taking the blood pressure of a pregnant woman. Reproduced from Petrie J, O'Brien E, Littler W, de Swiet M, Padfield P, Coats A, Mee F. CD-rom on Blood Pressure Measurement. BMJ Publications, 1998

21

Part II: Conventional sphygmomanometry

Basic requirements for auscultatory measurement of blood pressure

The century old technique of Riva Rocci/Korotkoff is now recognised to be fraught with inaccuracies that may lead to the misdiagnosis of abnormal blood pressure in many people. As a result, the auscultatory technique is being replaced by automated techniques, and its place in medicine may soon be of historical rather than practical interest. Measurement of blood pressure in clinical practice is dependent on the accurate transmission and interpretation of a signal (the Korotkoff sound or pulse wave) from a patient through a device (the sphygmomanometer) to an observer. Errors in measurement can occur at any interaction point during the technique, but the observer is by far the most fallible component.

Observer error

The major cause of observer error is the variability of blood pressure and the misleading measurements that constitute the phenomenon of white coat hypertension and masked hypertension now may be added to this list. Training of observers in the technique of auscultatory measurement of blood pressure is often taken for granted. Instruction to medical students and nurses has not always been as comprehensive as it might be, and assessment for competence in the measurement of blood pressure has been a relatively recent development. A number of training methods exist.

Mercury and aneroid sphygmomanometers

The mercury sphygmomanometer is a reliable device, but all too often its continuing efficiency has been taken for granted. Aneroid manometers are not as accurate. These two types of device have certain features in common; these are:

Inflation-deflation system
The inflation-deflation system consists of an inflating and deflating mechanism connected by rubber tubing to an occluding bladder. The standard mercury and aneroid sphygmomanometers used in clinical practice are operated manually, with inflation by means of a bulb compressed by hand and deflation by means of a release valve, which is also controlled by hand. The pump and control valve are connected to the inflatable bladder and to the sphygmomanometer. One of the most common sources of error in sphygmomanometers is the control valve.

Mercury sphygmomanometers
The mercury sphygmomanometer is a simple and accurate device that can be serviced easily, but concerns rightly exist about the toxicity of mercury for people who use mercury sphygmomanometers and those who service them. The greatest concern about mercury, however, is its toxic effect on the environment, and mercury increasingly is being banned from use in medicine.

Aneroid sphygmomanometers
Aneroid sphygmomanometers register pressure through a bellows and lever system that is more intricate mechanically than the mercury reservoir and column. The jolts and bumps of

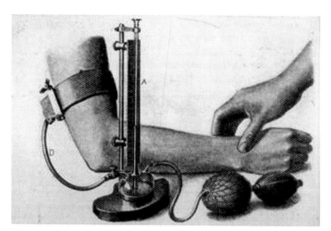

Riva-Rocci sphygmomanometer. Reproduced from O'Brien E, Fitzgerald D. The history of indirect blood pressure measurement. In: *Blood pressure measurement*, O'Brien E, O'Malley K, eds. Amsterdam: Elsevier, 1991

Observer influences

- Systematic error—intraobserver and interobserver error
- Terminal digit preference—rounding off to favoured digit, usually 0
- Observer prejudice—choice of measured pressure influenced by what observer wishes it to be
- White coat hypertension—high office and normal daytime ambulatory blood pressure
- Masked hypertension—normal office and high daytime ambulatory blood pressure

Training methods

- Direct instruction with a binaural or multiaural stethoscope
- Manuals, booklets and guidelines
- Audiotapes, CD-Rom, and DVD with instruction and visual falling mercury column and Korotkoff sounds permitting assessment of competence

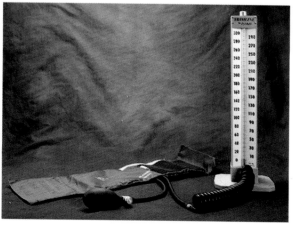

Mercury sphygmomanometer

Features and weaknesses common to mercury and aneroid sphygmomanometers

Features
- Inflation-deflation system
- Occluding bladder encased in a cuff
- Auscultation of Korotkoff sounds with stethoscope
- Connecting rubber tubing

Weaknesses
- Defective control valve—leakage:
    —Underestimation of systolic blood pressure
    —Overestimation of diastolic blood pressure
- Leaks as a result of cracked or perished rubber:
    —Mercury fall cannot be controlled
- Inadequate tubing:
    —Minimum length of 70 cm between cuff and manometer
    —Minimum length of 30 cm between pump and cuff
- Connections not airtight

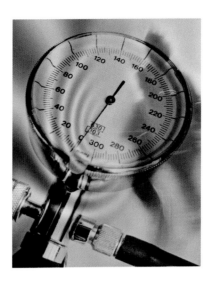

Aneroid gauge. With permission from Miriam Maslo/Science Photo Library

everyday use affect accuracy over time, which usually leads to falsely low readings and thus underestimations of blood pressure. They are therefore less accurate in use than mercury sphygmomanometers. Moreover, aneroid sphygmomanometry is also prone to all the problems of the auscultatory technique. As mercury sphygmomanometers are removed from clinical practice, people tend to replace them with aneroid devices on the false assumption that they are equally accurate. Remarkably little literature exists on the accuracy of aneroid devices and what does is generally negative (see www.dableducational.org).

Stethoscope
A stethoscope should be of high quality, with clean and well fitting earpieces. Whether the bell or diaphragm is used in routine measurement of blood pressure probably does not matter much, as long as the stethoscope is placed over the palpated brachial artery in the antecubital fossa. As the diaphragm covers a larger area and is easier to hold than a bell endpiece, it is reasonable to recommend it for routine clinical measurement of blood pressure.

Maintenance

To check and maintain mercury sphygmomanometers is easy, but great care should be taken when mercury is handled. Mercury sphygmomanometers need cleaning and checking at least every six months in hospital use and every 12 months in general use. In practice, doctors often neglect to have sphygmomanometers checked and serviced. The responsibility for reporting faulty equipment or lack of appropriate cuffs lies with the observer, who should always refuse to use defective or inappropriate equipment.

Aneroid sphygmomanometers should be checked every six months against an accurate mercury sphygmomanometer over the entire pressure range. This can be done by connecting the aneroid sphygmomanometer via a Y piece to the tubing of the mercury sphygmomanometer and inflating the cuff around a bottle or cylinder. If inaccuracies or other faults are found, the instrument must be repaired by the manufacturer or supplier.

Alternative devices to mercury sphygmomanometers

Non-automated devices
Oscillometric measurement of blood pressure has a number of inherent limitations. It is therefore unlikely to be accepted as the gold standard for conventional measurement of blood pressure.

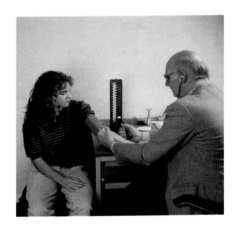

Placement of stethoscope. With permission from Sheila Terry/Science Photo Library

Accuracy limits
- Difference in accuracy of aneroid *v* mercury sphygmomanometer <3 mm Hg
- Surveys have shown:
    —58% aneroid devices have errors >4 mm Hg
    —30% aneroid devices have errors >7 mm Hg
    —50% hospital sphygmomanometers are defective
- Maintenance policy is mandatory but rarely in place

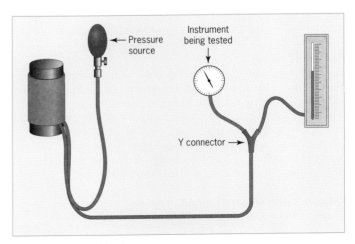

Calibration of aneroid sphygmomanometer

Alternative devices to the mercury sphygmomanometer, which combine the features of electronic and mercury devices by using an electronic pressure gauge as a substitute for the mercury column, are now being produced. These devices, which are known as "hybrid" sphygmomanometers, display cuff pressure as a simulated mercury column with an array of liquid crystal displays and as a digital readout on a liquid crystal display. The cuff is deflated in the normal way; when systolic and diastolic pressure are heard, a button next to the deflation knob is pressed, which freezes the digital display to show systolic and diastolic pressures. This offers the potential of eliminating terminal digit preference, which is a major problem with the clinical use of any auscultatory monitor. The observer is therefore able to measure blood pressure with the traditional auscultatory technique without necessarily having to rely on automated readings. This is achieved without the problems associated with mercury columns or aneroid devices.

Automated devices
As technology improves, mercury and aneroid devices will soon be replaced by accurate automated sphygmomanometers.

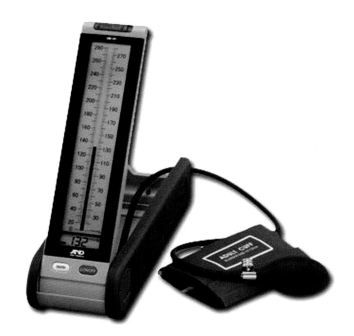

Mercury-free sphygmomanometer

Advantages and disadvantages of automated devices

Advantages

- Provide printouts with:
  —Systolic and diastolic blood pressure
  —Mean blood pressure
  —Heart rate
  —Time of measurement
  —Date of measurement
- Eliminate observer error
- Eliminate observer bias
- Eliminate observer digit preference
- Minimal training needed
- Store data for future analysis and comparision
- Ability to plot trends

Disadvantages

- Poor record for accuracy but improving
- Designed for self measurement rather than clinical use
- All use oscillometric measurement
  —Point of maximal cuff oscillation—mean blood pressure
  —Systolic and diastolic blood pressure derived from algorithm
  —Details of algorithm known only to manufacturer
- Oscillometric technique fails in some individuals
- Oscillometric technique not accurate in rapid atrial fibrillation

---

Performing auscultatory measurements

Position of manometer
The observer should take care to position the manometer so that the scale can be read easily. Accurate measurement is achieved most effectively with stand mounted models, which can easily be adjusted to suit the height of the observer. The mercury manometer has a vertical scale, and errors will occur unless the eye is kept close to the level of the meniscus. The aneroid scale is a composite of vertical and horizontal divisions and numbers, and it must be viewed straight on, with the eye on a line perpendicular to the centre of the face of the gauge.

Placement of cuff
The cuff should be wrapped around the arm, ensuring that the dimensions of the bladder are accurate. If the bladder does not completely encircle the arm, its centre must be over the brachial artery. The rubber tubes from the bladder are usually placed inferiorly, often at the site of the brachial artery, but placing them superiorly allows easy access to the antecubital fossa for auscultation. The lower edge of the cuff should be 2–3 cm above the point of brachial artery pulsation.

Palpatory estimation of blood pressure
The brachial artery should be palpated while the cuff is inflated rapidly to about 30 mm Hg above the point where the pulse disappears; the cuff is then deflated slowly, and the observer notes the pressure at which the pulse reappears.

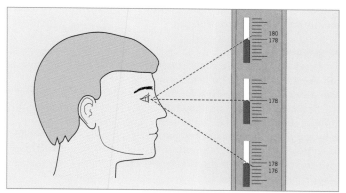

Eye level

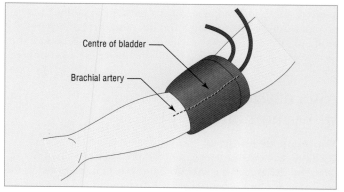

Placement of cuff

This is the approximate level of the systolic pressure. Palpatory estimation is important, because phase I sounds sometimes disappear as pressure is reduced and reappear at a lower level (the auscultatory gap), which results in systolic pressure being underestimated unless already determined by palpation. The palpatory technique is useful in patients in whom auscultatory endpoints may be difficult to judge accurately, for example, pregnant women, patients in shock, and those who are exercising. (The radial artery is often used for palpatory estimation of the systolic pressure but use of the brachial artery also allows the observer to establish its location before auscultation begins.)

Diastolic dilemma
For many years recommendations on blood pressure measurement have been uncertain about the diastolic end-point—the so called diastolic dilemma. Phase IV (muffling) may coincide with or be as much as 10 mm Hg higher than phase V (disappearance), but usually the difference is less than 5 mm Hg. Disappearance of sounds (phase V) should be taken as diastolic pressure. When the Korotkoff sounds persist down to zero, muffling of sounds (phase IV) should be recorded for diastolic pressure, and a note made to this effect.

Recording blood pressure
To make measurement of conventional blood pressure more informative and accurate, it is important to record the circumstances of measurement as well as the levels of blood pressure recorded. Reliability of measurement is improved if repeated measurements are made and measurement of ambulatory blood pressure or self-measurement of blood pressure, or both, give much valuable information that cannot be obtained with measurement of conventional blood pressure.

Points to be noted
- Measurements should be noted to the nearest single mm Hg, without rounding off to the nearest 5 or 10 mm Hg
- Note state of patient—anxious or relaxed
- Note position of patient for measurement—lying, sitting, or standing
- Note arm (right or left) in which blood pressure is measured; readings should be taken in both arms at the first visit
- Note arm circumference
- Note inflatable bladder dimensions
- Identify Korotkoff phases IV and V for diastolic pressure
- Note presence of auscultatory gap
- Note time of drug ingestion, if appropriate
- At least two measurements should be taken at each visit at intervals of at least one minute

Korotkoff sounds
- **Phase I**—the first appearance of faint, repetitive, clear tapping sounds that gradually increase in intensity for at least two consecutive beats is the systolic blood pressure
- **Phase II**—a brief period may follow phase I, during which the sounds soften and acquire a swishing quality
- **Auscultatory gap**—in some patients, sounds may disappear altogether for a short time
- **Phase III**—the return of sharper sounds that become crisper to regain, or even exceed, the intensity of the sound in phase I. The clinical significance, if any, of phases II and III has not been established
- **Phase IV**—the distinct abrupt muffling of sounds, which become soft and blowing in quality
- **Phase V**—the point at which all sounds finally disappear completely is the diastolic pressure

Manometer position
- Manometer <3 feet from observer
- Mercury column should be vertical
- Mercury column at eye level—standard mounted models can be adjusted to suit the height of the observer
- Observer's eye should follow the level of the mercury meniscus
- Aneroid scale must be viewed straight on with eye on a line perpendicular to the centre of the face of the gauge

Steps in measurement
- Place the stethoscope gently over the brachial artery at the point of maximal pulsation
- Hold stethoscope firmly and evenly but without excessive pressure—excess pressure may distort artery and produce sounds below diastolic pressure
- Stethoscope end-piece should not touch clothing, cuff, or rubber tubes to avoid friction sounds
- Inflate cuff rapidly to about 30 mm Hg above palpated systolic pressure
- Deflate cuff at a rate of 2 to 3 mm Hg per pulse beat (or per second) during which the Korotkoff sounds will be heard
- Deflate cuff rapidly after all sounds disappear
- Make sure cuff is completely deflated before repeating measurement so as to avoid venous congestion of the arm

Part III: Ambulatory blood pressure measurement

Ambulatory blood pressure measurement is used increasingly in clinical practice. The evidence that it gives information over and above measurement of conventional blood pressure has been increasing steadily over the past 25 years. Ambulatory blood pressure measurement is now accepted internationally as an indispensable investigation in patients with established and suspected hypertension.

Choosing devices and software

The first step in adopting ambulatory blood pressure measurement is to select an accurate device (see www.dableducational.org for the latest selection of accurate devices). Ambulatory blood pressure measurement in clinical practice is simplified by a standardised graphical presentation of the recording (much as is the case for electrocardiograph recordings) regardless of the type of monitor used. This saves the user having to become familiar with a variety of programs and simplifies the interchange of recordings between hospitals and primary care practices. Interpretive reports provide help for doctors and nurses unfamiliar with the technique, and the time needed for a doctor to report on each measurement is reduced, which lessens the cost of the technique.

Financial considerations

Analysis of the cost-benefit of ambulatory blood pressure measurement is complex and awaits full study. It is more expensive than measurement of conventional blood pressure, but the evidence strongly suggests benefits to patients justify the additional expense.

Training requirements

Measurement of ambulatory blood pressure is a specialised technique and should be approached with the care reserved for any such procedure. An understanding of the principles of the measurement of conventional blood pressure, cuff fitting, monitor function, and analysis and interpretation of the data produced is needed. In practice, a nurse with an interest and experience in hypertension can master the use of devices to measure ambulatory blood pressure after relatively little training. Analysis and interpretation of profiles for ambulatory blood pressure, however, need experience in the technique; this is achieved best by the doctor in charge of a service that provides ambulatory blood pressure measurement.

Using a monitor

Time needs to be allowed to fit the monitor and prepare the patient for the monitoring period if good results are to be obtained. The key to successful measurement of ambulatory blood pressure is educating the patient on the process of monitoring, and the instructions should be explained and printed on a diary card. Blood pressures recorded during the 24 hours can be analysed in a number of ways, which can be selected in the software program. One simple and popular method is to assess the time of awakening and sleeping from entries in diary cards. Another method uses fixed times, in which the retiring period (2101 to 0059) and rising period

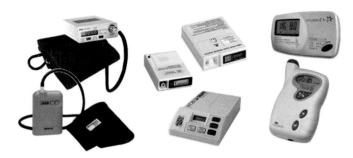

Selection of devices to measure ambulatory blood pressure

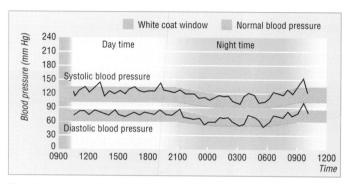

Plot of normal ambulatory blood pressure. Plot generated by dabl ABPM—© dabl 2006 (www.dabl.ie)

Financial considerations in measurement of ambulatory blood pressure

Against
- Devices remain expensive but are becoming cheaper
- Staff need to be trained on the use and interpretation of data
- Staff need to fit monitors, instruct patients, and download data from recorders

In favour
- Identifies patients with white coat hypertension and masked hypertension
- Reduces drug prescribing
- Helps decision making for insurance proposals
- Helps decision making for employers
- Shows efficacy of treatment
    —More efficient prescribing of drugs
    —Decreased prescribing of drugs
- Identifies patients with nocturnal hypertension at high risk of stroke
- Predicts outcome more accurately than other blood pressure measurements

---

Using a monitor to measure ambulatory blood pressure
- 15–30 minutes needed
- Patient should be relaxed in quiet room
- Enter patient details into monitor
- Measure blood pressure in each arm
    —If difference in systolic blood pressure <10 mm Hg, use non-dominant arm
    —If difference in systolic blood pressure ≥10 mm Hg, use higher pressure arm
- Select appropriate cuff
- Select frequency of measurement—usually every 30 minutes day and night
- Inactivate liquid crystal display
- Give patient written instructions and a diary card
- Instruct patient on how to remove and inactivate monitor after 24 hours

(0601 to 0859; during which blood pressure is subject to considerable variation) are eliminated. The daytime period lasts from 0900 to 2100 and the night-time period from 0100 to 0600. In this way, variations between young and old people and between people of different cultures are eliminated, to some extent, from the analysis.

The reproducibility of measurements of ambulatory blood pressure is improved when the measurements are taken on like days—for example, working days or recreational days. A diary card may be used to record symptoms and events that could influence ambulatory blood pressure measurement.

Editing data

Many statistical techniques exist to describe different aspects of ambulatory records, and no one method is ideal. If sufficient measurements are available, editing is not needed to calculate average values for 24 hours, daytime, and night-time. Only grossly incorrect readings should be deleted from recordings.

Normal levels

As with the measurement of conventional blood pressure, normal ranges for ambulatory blood pressures have been the subject of much debate over the years. General agreement is that levels of ambulatory blood pressure are appreciably lower than normal levels for conventional blood pressure.

Clinical indications

Ambulatory blood pressure measurement provides a large number of measurements over a period of time, usually 24 hours, which can be plotted to give a profile of the behaviour of a person's blood pressure. In practice, although the average daytime or night-time values from ambulatory blood pressure measurement are used to make decisions, the clinical use of ambulatory blood pressure has identified a number of phenomena in hypertension.

Suspected white coat hypertension

White coat hypertension, or isolated office hypertension, is present in people who seem to have hypertension from measurement of conventional blood pressure but have normal ambulatory blood pressure. The most popular definition of white coat hypertension requires:

- blood pressure measured by conventional techniques in the office, clinic, or surgery >140/90 mm Hg on at least three occasions
- normal ambulatory blood pressure throughout the 24 hours, except for the first hour, when the patient is under the pressor influence of the medical environment while having the monitor fitted.

White coat hypertension is present in 10–20% of clinic referrals for ambulatory blood pressure measurement; the reported prevalence in the population is around 10%. Patients with high conventional blood pressure and normal average daytime ambulatory pressures have a higher risk of major cardiovascular events than those with clinically normal blood pressure and a lower risk than those with high pressures during the daytime. White coat hypertension may affect young people, elderly people, people with normal blood pressure, those with hypertension, and pregnant women.

White coat effect

White coat hypertension should be distinguished from white coat effect, which is the term used to describe the increase in

Recommended normal levels for ambulatory blood pressure in adults*

Status	Blood pressure (mm Hg)		
	Optimal	Normal	Abnormal
Awake	< 130/80	< 135/85	> 140/90
Asleep	< 115/65	< 120/70	> 125/75

*Normal and abnormal demarcation levels based on evidence from several studies. Evidence not available to make recommendations for intermediate pressure ranges between normal and abnormal levels or for recommendations lower than those given. The levels are only a guide to normality, and lower optimal levels may be more appropriate in patients whose total profile of cardiovascular risk factors is high, and those with comorbid disease such as diabetes.

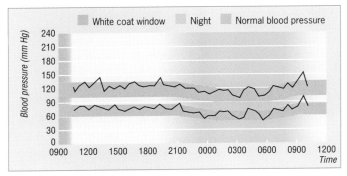

Normal ambulatory blood pressure monitoring pattern—On the basis of the data recorded and the available literature, the ambulatory blood pressure monitoring pattern suggests normal 24-hour systolic and diastolic blood pressure (128/78 mm Hg daytime, 110/62 mm Hg night-time). Plot and report generated by dabl ABPM—© dabl 2006 (www.dabl.ie)

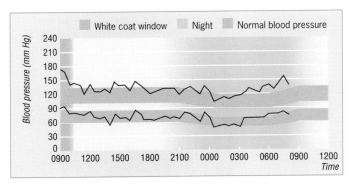

White coat hypertension—On the basis of the data recorded and the available literature, the ambulatory blood pressure monitoring pattern suggests white coat hypertension (175/95 mm Hg) with otherwise normal 24-hour systolic and diastolic blood pressure (133/71 mm Hg daytime, 119/59 mm Hg night-time). Plot and report generated by dabl ABPM—© dabl 2006 (www.dabl.ie)

pressure that occurs in the medical environment regardless of the daytime ambulatory blood pressure. It is present in most patients with hypertension, who usually tend to have conventional blood pressures higher than the average daytime ambulatory blood pressure, which is still higher than normal.

Masked hypertension (isolated ambulatory hypertension)

Recently, patients in whom conventional blood pressure is normal but ambulatory blood pressure is high have been identified. Because ambulatory blood pressure gives a better classification of risk than conventional blood pressure, these people should be regarded genuinely as being hypertensive and at risk. The problem for doctors in clinical practice is how to identify and manage these patients, who may number as many as 10 million people in the United States.

Resistant hypertension

Ambulatory blood pressure may be useful in patients with resistant hypertension (conventional blood pressure consistently >150/90 mm Hg despite treatment with three antihypertensive drugs). It may indicate that the apparent lack of response is the result of the white coat phenomenon.

Elderly patients in whom treatment is being considered

A number of patterns of ambulatory blood pressure may be found in elderly people. Conventional systolic blood pressure in elderly people may be an average of 20 mm Hg higher than daytime ambulatory blood pressure. A number of hypotensive states as a result of baroreceptor or autonomic failure are common in elderly people. As elderly people particularly can be susceptible to the adverse effects of drugs used to reduce blood pressure, identification of hypotension becomes especially important, although its management may present a considerable therapeutic challenge.

Isolated diastolic hypertension

High diastolic blood pressure with normal systolic ambulatory blood pressure increasingly is being recognised. The importance of isolated diastolic hypertension awaits further research.

Suspected nocturnal hypertension

Ambulatory blood pressure measurement allows blood pressure to be measured during sleep. Recent evidence showed that people whose blood pressure remains high at night (non-dippers) rather than falling below daytime levels (as in most people) are at higher risk of stroke, heart attack, and cardiovascular death. The pattern of non-dipping may provide

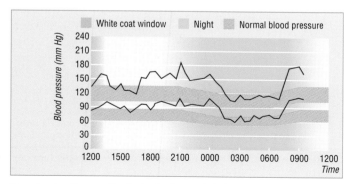

Hypertensive dipper—On the basis of recorded data and available literature, ambulatory blood pressure suggests mild daytime systolic and diastolic hypertension (147/93 mm Hg) and normal night-time systolic and diastolic blood pressure (111/66 mm Hg) with white coat effect (158/90 mm Hg). Plot and report generated by dabl ABPM—© dabl 2006 (www.dabl.ie)

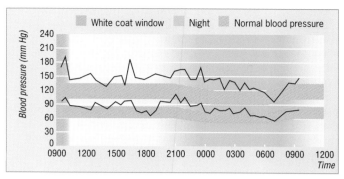

White coat effect—On the basis of the data recorded and the available literature, the pattern suggests mild daytime systolic hypertension (149 mm Hg), borderline daytime diastolic hypertension (87 mm Hg), borderline night-time systolic hypertension (121 mm Hg), and normal night-time diastolic blood pressure (67 mm Hg) with white coat effect (187/104 mm Hg). Plot and report generated by dabl ABPM—© dabl 2006 (www.dabl.ie)

Factors suspicious for masked hypertension

- High conventional blood pressure recorded at some time
- Normal or normal-high conventional blood pressure and early left ventricular hypertrophy in a young patient
- Family history of hypertension in two parents
- Multiple risks for cardiovascular disease
- Diabetes

Patterns of ambulatory blood pressure in elderly people

- White coat hypertension (common)
- Masked hypertension
- Isolated systolic hypertension (most common)
- Nocturnal hypertension
- Autonomic or baroreceptor failure (daytime hypotension or nocturnal hypertension)
- Postural hypotension
- Drug induced hypotension
- Post-prandial hypotension

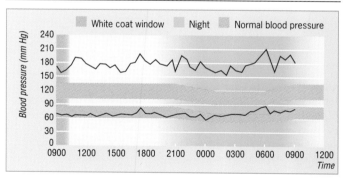

Isolated systolic hypertension—On the basis of recorded data and available literature, the pattern suggests severe 24-hour isolated systolic hypertension (176/68 mm Hg daytime, 169/70 mm Hg night-time). Plot and report generated by dabl ABPM—© dabl 2006 (www.dabl.ie)

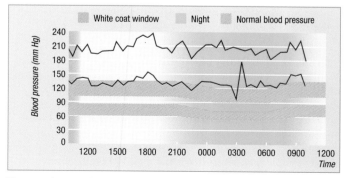

Hypertensive non-dipper—On the basis of recorded data and available literature, the pattern suggests severe systolic and diastolic hypertension over 24 hours (209/135 mm Hg daytime and 205/130 mm Hg at night). Plot and report generated by dabl ABPM—© dabl 2006 (www.dabl.ie)

a useful (although non-specific) clue to the presence of secondary hypertension.

Pregnancy

As in the non-pregnant state, the main use for ambulatory blood pressure measurement in pregnancy is to identify white coat hypertension, which may occur in nearly 30% of pregnant women. Its recognition is important, so that pregnant women are not admitted to hospital or given antihypertensive drugs unnecessarily or excessively. Normal values for ambulatory blood pressure in the pregnant population are available, and changes in pressure, which occur during the trimesters of pregnancy and the postpartum period, have been defined.

Type I diabetes

In people with type I diabetes, a blunted or absent drop in blood pressure from day to night is an even more serious predictor for increased cardiovascular complications than in patients with hypertension without diabetes. The aim of antihypertensive drugs should be to achieve lower levels of blood pressure in diabetic than in non-diabetic patients.

Ambulatory hypotension

Ambulatory blood pressure measurement is helpful in identifying hypotensive episodes in elderly people, but it also may be used in young patients in whom hypotension is suspected as a cause of symptoms. Ambulatory blood pressure measurement may also show drug induced decreases in blood pressure in patients being treated for hypertension.

Who should be monitored

Ambulatory blood pressure measurement may be inconvenient to patients and should be used, therefore, with discretion. The decision as to when to repeat ambulatory blood pressure measurement is largely one of clinical judgment. The frequency of repeat ambulatory blood pressure measurement must be guided by the response to treatment, the stability of blood pressure control, and the overall cardiovascular risk profile. Where the risk for cardiovascular complications is high, the frequency is more than justified by the need for tight blood pressure control, whereas when the risk is low, less frequent measurement is needed. Self-measurement of blood pressure may be combined with ambulatory blood pressure measurement to reduce the frequency of the latter.

Indications for re-monitoring for ambulatory blood pressure measurement

- Subjects with white coat hypertension
- Treated patients with major white coat effect
- Elderly patients with symptoms suggesting orthostatic hypotension
- Patients with nocturnal hypertension
- To compare effect of changes in medication
- High-risk patients
- Diabetic patients

Mean (SD) ambulatory blood pressures during pregnancy

Gestation (weeks)	Blood pressure (mm Hg)			
	Daytime		Night-time	
	Systolic	Diastolic	Systolic	Diastolic
9–16	115 (8)	70 (7)	100 (7)	55 (5)
18–24	115 (8)	69 (6)	99 (8)	54 (6)
26–32	116 (9)	70 (7)	101 (8)	55 (6)
33–40	119 (9)	74 (7)	106 (8)	58 (7)

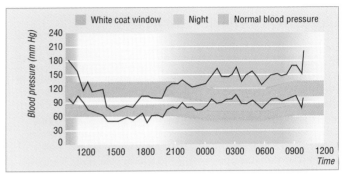

Ambulatory hypotension—On the basis of recorded data and available literature, ambulatory blood pressure monitoring pattern suggests low daytime systolic blood pressure (100 mm Hg) and normal daytime diastolic blood pressure (61 mm Hg) and moderate night-time systolic and diastolic hypertension (146/89 mm Hg) with white coat effect (200/102 mm Hg). Plot and report generated by dabl ABPM—© dabl 2006 (www.dabl.ie)

The role of ambulatory blood pressure in guiding drug treatment is the subject of much research, but recent reviews have highlighted the potential of ambulatory blood pressure measurement over 24 hours in guiding the use of antihypertensive drugs

---

Ambulatory blood pressure measurement as a guide to drug treatment

- Efficacy of treatment in patients with white coat effect
- Efficacy of treatment over 24 hours—especially during the night
- Shows excessive effects of drugs matched to occurrence of symptoms
- Shows drug induced hypotension

Suggested frequency for repeat ambulatory blood pressure measurement

- White coat hypertension pattern—confirm diagnosis in 3–6 months
- White coat pattern and low risk profile—repeat ambulatory blood pressure measurement every 1 to 2 years
- White coat hypertension pattern and high risk profile—repeat ambulatory blood pressure measurement every 6 months to detect possible transition to sustained hypertension requiring treatment
- To determine efficacy of treatment
  —If low risk and controlled without target organ damage—annual ambulatory blood pressure measurement
  —If high risk and/or poorly controlled with target organ damage—more frequent ambulatory blood pressure measurement

Part IV: Self-measurement of blood pressure

For more than 50 years, self-measured blood pressures in the home have been recognised to be lower than those recorded by a doctor. Self-measurement is popular with the public, as evidenced by the huge sales of devices for self-monitoring. Doctors have tended to be cautious in their use of the technique, but interest in self-measurement of blood pressure is reviving, although the fact that much research is needed is recognised.

General considerations

Devices and validation

Monitors for self-measurement of blood pressure include mercury column sphygmomanometers, aneroid manometers, and electronic semi-automatic or automatic devices. The sale of electronic devices designed for self-measurement of blood pressure is not necessarily subject to any medical influence. This freedom from medical control, coupled with a growing public desire to know more about health and illness, has resulted in the manufacture and marketing of a vast array of such devices, few of which have been evaluated according to the procedures considered necessary for equipment used to measure blood pressure in clinical practice.

Automated devices available for self-measurement all use the oscillometric technique. Three categories are available: devices that measure blood pressure in the upper arm, wrist, or finger.

Lack of popularity for self-measurement

- Patients need to be trained in the technique
- Technique subject to bias by patients (can be overcome with printouts from device)
- May cause anxiety to certain patients
- May make some patients obsessive about levels of blood pressure
- Devices largely have not been validated
- Most devices have been inaccurate (this is changing for the better)
- Lack of evidence to support use of the technique
- Not suitable for patients with certain disabilities

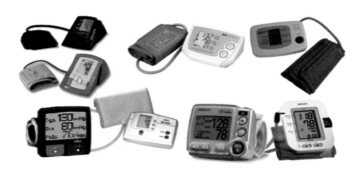

Selection of devices for self-measurement of blood pressure

Accuracy of wrist devices for self-measurement of blood pressure

Device	AAMI	BHS	ESH	Circumstance	Recommendation
Braun PrecisionSensor BP2000	Pass			At rest, manufacturer assistance	Questionable
Braun PrecisionSensor BP2550	Pass	B/B		Recruitment violation (AAMI) Recruitment violation and analysis errors (BHS)	Questionable
		B/B		Abstract, results of systolic pressure unclear	Questionable
Braun PrecisionSensor BP2550(UG)			Pass/pass	At rest	Recommended
Braun VitalScan	Pass			Abstract; version not stated	Questionable
Braun VitalScan Plus 1650		Pass		Abstracts	Questionable
Omron 637IT	Pass	B/A	Fail/pass	Abstract; BHS 'pass' incorrectly reported Ad hoc protocol, with or without position sensor, standard protocol projections inconclusive	Questionable Questionable

AAMI = American Association of Medical Instrumentation; BHS = British Hypertension Society; ESH = European Society for Hypertension. Table adapted from dabl® Educational Trust.

User procedure

The same principles apply to self-measurement as apply to measurement in general. Some points, however, need emphasis.

Use in primary care

At present, self-measurement of blood pressure is performed mostly by patients on their own initiative, with devices bought on the free market without medical control. Primary care doctors should see self-measurement as a means of gaining further insight into control of blood pressure and the effects of management strategies in motivated and informed patients who remain under medical supervision.

The website dableducational shows the latest selection of accurate devices for self-measurement. See example table—for full details go to www.dableducational.org

Advantages of current devices for self-measurement

- Inexpensive
- Remove observer bias
- Eliminate terminal digit preference
- Potential to provide printouts of data or store data:
  - —Levels of systolic and diastolic blood pressures
  - —Mean blood pressure
  - —Heart rate
  - —Time and date of measurements
  - —Trend plots
- Potential to provide electronic storage and transmission of data

Frequency and timing of self-measurement

The frequency of self-measurement may vary according to the indication and the information that is sought. Frequent measurement may be recommended for individual patients (such as those with poor compliance) or for participants in pharmacological studies.

Diagnostic thresholds

The threshold level of 135/85 mm Hg for self-measurement of blood pressure is the same as that for mean daytime ambulatory blood pressure.

Clinical indications

The clinical applications of self-measurement of blood pressure are beginning to become apparent only as the technique is used more widely and scientific data is gathered.

White coat hypertension

Self-measurement has been proposed as a useful alternative to measurement of ambulatory blood pressure to detect white coat hypertension. The finding of normal blood pressure on self-measurement, however, does not rule out the possibility that the blood pressure may be higher at other times of the day. Self-measurement, which is less costly and more convenient than measurement of ambulatory pressure, may be appropriate for long term follow up of patients with white coat hypertension.

Guiding antihypertensive treatment

Self-measurement may have a role in assessing the response to antihypertensive drug treatment outside the medical environment and over time. Measurement of blood pressure in the home environment under similar everyday conditions avoids the white coat effect and reduces variability. Self-measurement can improve the assessment of blood pressure control in the management of hypertension and clinical trials. Recent systematic reviews have shown that self monitoring improves blood pressure control. Whether or not this is through improved adherence to drug treatment, by improved tailoring of drug treatment or by other methods is not fully established.

Elderly patients

Feasibility of self-measurement in elderly patients may be influenced by physical and intellectual limitations and the complexity of the chosen device. Studies in elderly people have shown that automatic equipment is more precise and easier to use than semi-automatic equipment.

Pregnancy

As in the general population, blood pressures recorded by self-measurement are lower than conventional blood pressures. Self-measurement may be useful for the diagnosis of white coat responders and to monitor the effect of antihypertensive drugs. Data storage and electronic transmission of data may have a particular role for patients who live at distance from the maternity clinic. Very few data are available, however, on levels of normality for self-measured blood pressure in the different stages of pregnancy and the use of the technique in pregnancy.

Points to consider for self-measurement

- Self-measurement should be performed after five minutes' rest
- Use devices that occlude brachial artery
- Wrist monitors unreliable but improving
- Finger monitors should not be used
- Device cuff must be at level of heart on arm with highest blood pressure
- Patient diaries may be unreliable
- Devices equipped with memory, with possibility of storing or transmitting data, preferred
- Readings from first day should be discarded
- Use all other data to calculate mean blood pressure
- In patients with arrhythmias, self-measurement may not be appropriate
- Self-measurement should be performed under medical supervision
- Patients should be trained in self-measurement and re-evaluated annually
- Self-measurement is suited to patients motivated towards the management of their own health

---

Scheme for self-measurement

Phase	Directions
Start	• Initial period of seven days • Two measurements between 0600 and 0900 • Two measurements between 1800 and 2100 • Discard readings from first day of measurement, which are unrepresentative because of anxiety and unfamiliarity • Use average measurements as reference for treatment and follow up
Treatment	• Repeat the above when the patient is on treatment • Morning measurements should be made before drugs are taken (trough levels of drug) • Average of two weeks on treatment should be compared with average of commencement phase to determine efficacy • Averages of two weeks on each treatment regimen should be compared to determine efficacy after a change in treatment
Follow-up	• Two measurements on one day a week in patients with good control of blood pressure • More frequent measurements in patients with poor control of blood pressure or compliance

---

Diagnostic thresholds for self-measurement

- Data from longitudinal studies limited
- Reference values derived principally from statistical evaluation of databases
- Suggested upper limit of normality 135/85 mm Hg (average of multiple readings taken on several days)
- Optimal 130/80 mm Hg (average of multiple readings taken on several days)

Factors that influence self-measurement

- Device accuracy—use only validated devices
- Observer prejudice (can be overcome with printouts and devices equipped with memory)
- Training of patients by doctors or nurses
- Training should focus on:
  —Use of device
  —Correct procedure
  —Interpretation of results
  —Need for maintenance and calibration
  —Essentials of hypertension
  —Management and treatment
- Seasonal variation (blood pressure is higher in winter and lower in summer)

Diabetes

Increasing evidence shows that stringent control of blood pressure reduces the cardiovascular and microvascular complications of diabetes. Self-measurement of blood pressure may be an additional means of ensuring that such control is achieved, although no data are available yet to guide the use of self-measurement in patients with diabetes.

Resistant hypertension

Patients with apparently uncontrolled blood pressure according to conventional monitoring may have adequate control at home. It may be possible to identify at least some of these patients by self-measurement, although ambulatory blood pressure is the preferred technique. In the evaluation of patients with resistant hypertension but no signs of target organ damage, the first step might be to use self-measurement; if the levels of blood pressure are low, measurement of ambulatory blood pressure may then be indicated to confirm the degree of control.

Predicting outcome

Self-measurement may offer some advantage over measurement of conventional blood pressure in predicting cardiovascular outcome in hypertension, but data are extremely limited and the results of ongoing trials are awaited. The results of cross sectional studies have shown that the degree of left ventricular hypertrophy determined by electrocardiography and echocardiography is correlated more strongly with self-measurement than conventional measurement.

Clinical indications for self-measurement

Accepted indications
- Screening for white coat hypertension
- Long term follow up
- Improving compliance to treatment
- Resistant hypertension

Potential indications
- Hypertension in pregnancy
- Hypertension in patients with diabetes
- Hypertension in elderly patients

Poor compliance with treatment

- One of the most important causes of refractory hypertension
- Self-measurement may provide patients with an understanding of high blood pressure and its response to treatment, thus improving compliance with treatment

5 Screening and management in primary care

G Y H Lip, D G Beevers

Patient involvement

The fourth guidelines of the British Hypertension Society (BHS 4) advocate the importance of patient involvement in the successful management and control of hypertension. This includes non-pharmacological or lifestyle changes, as well as patient involvement when considering drug treatment, including education about drugs patients should take and the drugs' proved benefits and possible side effects.

Patients also need to be warned that, on average, 75% of patients with hypertension need two or more drugs and that one third will need three or more drugs to achieve good control of blood pressure. The number of drugs needed may be even higher in patients with diabetes, in view of the lower thresholds for treatment in this group.

Many patients are keen to help with the management of their hypertension with home recording of blood pressure. Many high street chemists now sell inexpensive semi-automatic devices for the measurement of blood pressure, but as many of these have not been validated for accuracy, it is important to check this when purchasing a devise. Blood pressures measured at home probably resemble ambulatory blood pressures measured over 24 hours more closely than conventional pressures, and it is therefore a more reliable index of cardiovascular risk than casual clinical or office readings.

The Blood Pressure Association in the United Kingdom was set up specifically to provide information and support to people with high blood pressure. Cards that record blood pressure that are held by patients can improve compliance with treatment, particularly if the patient is attending a secondary referral clinic.

Health care systems
National service frameworks
The national service frameworks provides healthcare service standards in relation to various diseases and patient groups, such as coronary artery disease, elderly people, and patients with diabetes. These frameworks have led to targets of achievement that have broadly led to improvements in care.

> **Patients should be encouraged to buy their own blood pressure machines. For more information, see Chapter 4, Part IV**

Formulation of an individual management plan

- Acknowledge in consultations that patients' assessments of risk are determined primarily by emotions not facts—healthcare professionals should be competent and caring
- Explain the trade off between benefits and harms, but avoid purely descriptive terms of risk, such as "low risk"
- Show patients their total cardiovascular risk in the next 10 years on the colour charts in the *British National Formulary*
- Use a consistent denominator—for example, one in 100 and five in 100 rather than one in 100 and one in 20
- Use absolute not relative numbers
- Use visual aids whenever possible
- Use probabilities—for example, "three out of every 10 patients have a side effect from this drug" rather than "you have a 30% chance of a side effect from this drug"

HYPERTENSION COOPERATION CARD

Name: Thomas Smith   DOB: 16/02/48

Address: 47 High Street

Post Code: W27 9BU

General Practitioner: Dr Autrobus

Date diagnosed hypertensive: 16/02/03

Cigarette smoker: No/**Yes**   Quantity: 20/d

Advice:
(1) Avoid being overweight
(2) Moderate alcohol consumption
(3) Restrict salt intake
(4) Show this card to all doctors and nurses who look after you
(5) Always bring your labels when consulting your doctor or nurse
(6) Don't stop taking tablets unless advised to by your doctor or nurse
(7) Your target blood pressure is below 140/80 mm Hg

Date	16/2/03	19/3/03	17/5/03	21/7/03	19/10/03	17/11/03	12/1/04	6/5/04	19/8/04	27/11/04
B.P.1	172/106	170/100	168/100	152/92	156/94	154/90	138/84	136/82	132/84	134/82
PULSE	98	52								
B.P.2	168/98	168/98	172/98	148/90	152/92	152/94	134/80	132/78	135/85	128/80
URINE	NAD									
WEIGHT (kg / st lb)	84.2	84.0	82.1	81.6	82.0	82.2	84.0	82.4	81.0	80.2
DRUG 1 Bendrofluazide	/	/	Start 2.5mg	2.5mg	Stop	/	/	/	/	/
DRUG 2 Lisinopril	/	/	/	/	Start 10mg	Increase 20mg	20mg	20mg	20mg	20mg
DRUG 3	/	/	/	/	/	/	/	/	/	/
DRUG 4	/	/	/	/	/	/	/	/	/	/
DRUG 5	/	/	/	/	/	/	/	/	/	/
DRUG 6 Simvastatin	/	/	/	/	/	Start 10mg	10mg	Increase 20mg	20mg	
SERUM UREA	6.2	/	/	/	/	6.0	/	/	/	/
SERUM POTASSIUM	4.2	/	/	/	/	/	/	/	/	/
SERUM CHOLESTEROL	7.1	/	/	/	/	/	/	/	/	/
NEXT VISIT	1/12	2/12	2/12	3/12	1/12	2/12	3/12	3/12	3/12	3/12
DOCTOR'S SIGNATURE	RA	AO	RA	RA	RA	RA	RA	RA	RA	AO

Example of patient's hypertension cooperation card

The importance of prevention of cardiovascular disease is recognised, including the detection and treatment of hypertension. The framework is broadly consistent with the Joint British Societies' recommendations and the fourth guidelines of the British Hypertension Society. One exception is that the national service framework defines "high risk primary prevention" as "people without diagnosed [coronary heart disease] or other occlusive arterial disease but with a 10 year [coronary heart disease] risk >30%", which equates to a risk of cardiovascular disease over 10 years >40%. This confusion about the risk of coronary heart disease and the risk of cardiovascular disease is unfortunate, but most guideline committees now accept that total cardiovascular risk should be assessed (that is, including stroke and heart attack).

National Institute for Clinical Excellence
The guidelines of the National Institute for Clinical Excellence do not address when aspirin and statin drugs should be used to reduce the total burden of cardiovascular risk in people with high blood pressure. Optimal management of blood pressure needs assessment of these risk factors and a "package of care" of multifactorial intervention to reduce cardiovascular risk, including all risk factors and not just blood pressure.

Primary care
Most patients with hypertension are managed in primary care, and general practitioners and practice nurses are responsible for measurement of blood pressure and the detection, treatment, and control of hypertension. The management of millions of patients with hypertension can therefore be achieved only within primary healthcare.

Only a minority of patients with hypertension need to be referred to blood pressure clinics based in hospitals. The accurate detection, assessment, and treatment of patients with hypertension leads to considerable reductions in the rates of stroke and heart attack. Unfortunately, many patients with hypertension are not receiving the management they need.

Doctors also seem to overestimate their own compliance with current guidelines on hypertension, especially with regard to the proportion of patients who have adequately controlled blood pressure. This limited awareness may represent a barrier to successful implementation of management guidelines. In addition, doctors tend to underestimate the adverse effects of blood pressure and its treatment on their patient's quality of life.

Screening
Hypertension has been described as a "silent killer". It is usually asymptomatic, and, for this reason, many patients with hypertension are undetected unless special measures are taken. Ongoing screening for hypertension in asymptomatic patients can take place within the context of primary healthcare.

Between 70% and 80% of a practice's population will visit their general practitioner at least once in three years, and screening for hypertension can take place at the same time. This is "opportunistic screening." Blood pressure should therefore be checked in all patients who visit their general practitioner if they have not attended for more than 12 months.

Patients with blood pressures > 140/95 mm Hg should be advised that their blood pressures are not quite normal and recalled for re-examination a few weeks later. They should be assessed fully for cardiovascular risk according to the guidelines of the British Hypertension Society.

National service frameworks

Older people	**Diabetes**
• Important sections on stroke, primary and secondary prevention, and rehabilitation • By April 2004, every general practice was required to identify and treat patients at risk of stroke, including those with hypertension and atrial fibrillation • Hypertension was recognised as an important risk factor • Lifestyle and pharmaceutical interventions recommended to maintain blood pressure <140/85 mm Hg, consistent with current guidelines of the British Hypertension Society	• Standard 4 states that "all adults with diabetes shall receive high quality care throughout their lifetime, including support to optimise the control of their blood glucose, [blood pressure], and other risk factors for developing the complications of diabetes"

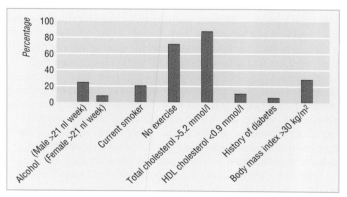

Concomitant risk factors in hypertension. HDL = high density lipoprotein

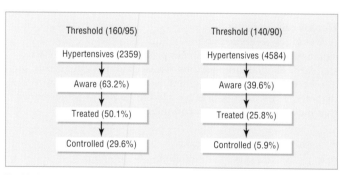

Health Survey for England 1994—proportions aware, treated, and controlled if thresholds for high blood pressure were 160/95 and 140/95 mm Hg

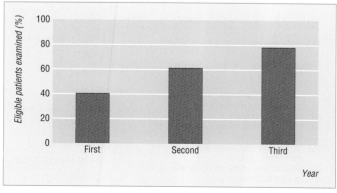

Screening for hypertension in primary care (opportunistic screening) in men aged 35–69 years in Scotland. Adapted from Barber et al. *BMJ* 1979;**1**:843–6

When screening for hypertension, certain "high risk" patient groups should be targeted specifically rather than waiting for them to attend for some other reason. This "selective" or "targeted" screening should be conducted in those at particular risk of developing hypertension or its vascular complications—for example, patients with diabetes.

In the primary care setting, high risk patients who stand to benefit most from control of blood pressure seem to be least likely to be controlled, despite being on a higher number of antihypertensive drugs. In one analysis, higher risk scores according to the Framingham study, female sex, diabetes, and impaired fasting glucose seemed to correlate negatively with control of blood pressure in primary care. Patients' knowledge of hypertension and the number of comorbid conditions seemed to correlate positively with control of blood pressure.

Specialist referral
About 10% of patients with hypertension in primary care have a secondary or underlying cause for their high blood pressure or may have very severe or resistant hypertension. Such patients should be referred for specialist assessment. Many general practitioners themselves have established dedicated hypertension clinics, which also can be run by appropriately trained nurse practitioners.

Current contract for general medical services for primary care (2003)
The current contract provides a major focus on quality of care and outcomes and rewards practices for delivering quality care to encourage even higher standards. Cardiovascular disease is covered, with standards related to coronary heart disease, stroke or transient ischaemic attacks, hypertension, and diabetes. These quality standards attract points that add to financial rewards to practices. Notably, 158 of the 550 clinical indicator points available relate directly to hypertension. This contract will hopefully increase focus on the detection, treatment, and quality of control of high blood pressure.

High risk patients who need targeted screening
- Pregnant women
- Patients with:
  - Strong family history of hypertension, heart attack, or stroke
  - Existing cardiovascular disease
  - Previous cardiovascular disease
  - Diabetes mellitus
  - Renal impairment
  - Systemic disease (including rheumatoid arthritis, polyarteritis, and systemic lupus erythematosus)
  - History of hypertension in pregnancy

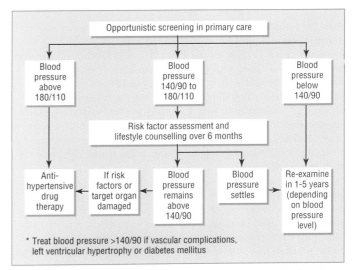

Triage or three box management of newly detected hypertension in primary cares setting. Patients with blood pressure ≥140/90 should be considered for ABPM to determine whether he or she has white coat hypertension

Hypertension quality indicators in new contract of the General Medical Service

Indicator	Points	Maximum threshold (%)
Secondary prevention in patients with chronic heart disease		
Ongoing management		
Percentage whose notes have record of blood pressure in past 15 months	7	90
Percentage whose latest blood pressure reading (measured in past 15 months) was ≤150/90 mm Hg	19	70
Patients with stroke or transient ischaemic attacks		
Ongoing management		
Percentage who have a record of blood pressure in the notes in past 15 months	2	90
Percentage whose latest blood pressure reading (measured in past 15 months) was ≤150/90 mm Hg	5	70
Patients with hypertension		
Records		
Practice can produce a register of patients with established hypertension	9	
Diagnosis and management		
Percentage whose notes record smoking status at least once	10	90
Percentage who smoke and whose notes contain a record that smoking cessation advice has been offered at least once	10	90
Ongoing management		
Percentage whose notes have a record of blood pressure in the past nine months	20	90
Percentage of patients whose latest blood pressure reading (measured in past nine months) was ≤150/90 mm Hg	56	70
Patients with diabetes mellitus		
Ongoing management		
Percentage whose notes have a record of blood pressure in the past 15 months	3	90
Percentage whose latest blood pressure is ≤145/85 mm Hg	17	55
Records and information about patients		
Blood pressure of patients aged ≥ 45 years is recorded in the preceding five years for at least 55% of patients	10	
Blood pressure of patients aged ≥ 45 years is recorded in the preceding five years for at least 75% of patients	5	

Hypertension and NHS resources

Heart and circulatory disease remain major causes of mortality in the United Kingdom. In 2002, cardiovascular disease caused 39% of deaths in the United Kingdom and killed just fewer than 238 000 people. Coronary heart disease, the main form of cardiovascular disease, causes more than 117 000 deaths a year in the United Kingdom; this equates to about one in five deaths in men and one in six deaths in women.

Importantly, 35% of premature deaths in men and 27% in women are from cardiovascular disease, which caused more than 67 000 premature deaths in the United Kingdom in 2002.

Important reductions in death rates for coronary heart disease and stroke have been seen since the late 1970s. Despite this, the United Kingdom has rates that are still among the highest in Western Europe. Death rates are higher in Scotland than the south of England, in manual workers than in non-manual workers, and in certain ethnic groups.

Although mortality from heart disease is falling rapidly, the morbidity associated with heart and circulatory disease is not decreasing. Recent estimates are that just fewer than 2.7 million people in the United Kingdom have coronary heart disease: about 1.51 million men who have or have had coronary heart disease (angina or heart attack) and about 1.16 million women. A general practitioner with a list of 2000 patients is estimated to have about 400 consultations each year for about 200 patients with hypertension.

Recent prescribing of drugs that affect blood pressure in England and Wales shows that the thiazides, β blockers, angiotensin converting enzyme inhibitors, and calcium channel blockers are used in similar quantities in primary care, although their costs vary by a factor of 10. The NHS writes more than about 90 million scripts annually, at a cost of £840 million; this is nearly 15% of the total annual cost of drugs in primary care.

The figure of concomitant risk factors is adapted from Poulter NR, et al., *Blood Pressure* 1996;5:209–15. The figure showing the results of the Health Survey for England 1994 is adapted from Colhoun H, et al. *J Hypertens* 1998;16:747–52. The figure showing screening for hypertension in primary care in men aged 35–69 years in Scotland is adapted from Barber JH, et al. *BMJ* 1979;1:843–6

The Blood Pressure Association is a UK charity dedicated to improving the prevention, detection, diagnosis, and treatment of high blood pressure. Their experts provide information on all aspects of the condition for people with high blood pressure and for health professionals (www.bpassoc.org.uk, tel: 020 8772 4994)

Use of drugs to reduce levels of blood pressure in primary care in England, 2001. Source: Department of Health

Drug class	Prescription items dispensed (000s)	Net cost of drug ingredients (£000s)*	Cost per prescription (£)[†]
Thiazides and related diuretics[‡]	16 092	22 672	1.41
Loop diuretics	10 519	16 534	1.57
Potassium sparing	1482	6055	4.09
Potassium sparing diuretics[‡] with other diuretics[‡]	3906	16 774	4.29
β Blockers[‡]	22 439	88 780	3.96
Vasodilator antihypertensive drugs	137	986	7.18
Centrally acting antihypertensive drugs	547	6687	12.22
Adrenergic neurone blocking drugs	3.6	88	24.85
Alpha adrenoceptor blocking drugs[‡]	3952	98 218	24.85
Angiotensin converting enzyme inhibitors[‡]	19 921	270 242	13.57
Angiotensin receptor blockers[‡]	5026	130 228	25.91
Calcium channel blockers[‡]	17 928	290 225	16.19
Total	101 953	947 489	9.29

*Before discounts and excluding dispensing costs.
[†]Net cost of drug ingredients divided by number of prescription items dispensed.
[‡]Drugs used regularly to treat essential hypertension.

6 Clinical assessment of patients with hypertension

G Y H Lip, D G Beevers

A full and careful clinical history is essential to assess the aetiology, causes, and complications of hypertension. Initial evaluation also should include measurement of total cardiovascular risk with the British Hypertension Society's colour charts. These charts are based on the Framingham equation, which calculates risk on the basis of routine characteristics (age and sex), smoking habit, levels of total and high density lipoprotein cholesterol, and blood pressure.

Symptoms

Most patients with uncomplicated hypertension are asymptomatic or present with non-specific (occasionally vague) symptoms. Most cases of hypertension are diagnosed as an incidental finding at a routine medical examination or after visiting the doctor for another condition.

The perception that patients with hypertension have frequent (and severe) headaches, epistaxis, and lethargy is a misconception. Even patients with severe hypertension may have no symptoms until they present with a vascular complication, such as myocardial infarction, stroke, or heart failure. When patients with hypertension are symptomatic, this is usually the result of anxiety and stress after diagnosis, "labelling," or the side effects of treatment.

Almost all patients with malignant hypertension are symptomatic, however, with visual deterioration or breathlessness as a result of heart failure. Headache is common but not universal, but many patients generally feel unwell, particularly if they have renal failure.

History

Attention should be directed to common associates of hypertension, such as diabetes mellitus, dyslipidaemia, and renal disease, as well as a past history of complications associated with hypertension. In women who present with hypertension, the obstetric history should be ascertained, including use of oral contraceptives, previous pre-eclampsia, or pregnancy induced hypertension.

Family history

Many patients with essential hypertension report a family history of hypertension. Any family history of coronary or cerebrovascular disease or premature vascular death should be determined, as this may help assess the patient's cardiovascular risk profile. Younger patients with hypertension and absolutely no family history need detailed investigations to detect possible underlying renal, renovascular, and adrenal causes of hypertension that are not familial. A family history of disease that may cause hypertension, such as autosomal dominant polycystic kidney disease, should be ascertained.

Drug history

Current or previous use of antihypertensive drugs should be assessed. Some drugs, such as oral contraceptives, may exacerbate hypertension. Drugs that cause sodium retention can exacerbate or impede control of hypertension and heart failure. Others may interact with antihypertensive drugs—for example, the effects of angiotensin converting enzyme inhibitors may be attenuated by non-steroidal anti-inflammatory drugs.

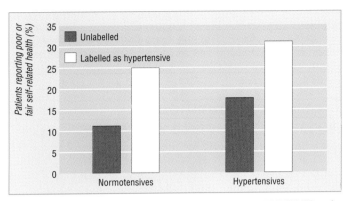

Diagnosis of hypertension and self-rated health from the NHANES III study. The trends are independent of age, ethnicity, gender, medication. Adapted from Barger SD, Muldoon MF. *J Human Hypertens* 2006;20:117–23

> Hypertension has been referred to as the "silent killer" because patients may have no symptoms until they present with a vascular complication

Hypertension induced by drugs

Cause	Examples
Drugs that cause sodium retention	Oral corticosteroids Adrenocorticotropic hormone Liquorice Carbenoxolone Indomethacin
Drugs that cause increased sympathetic activity	Ephedrine Cold cures Monoamine oxidase inhibitors
Direct vasoconstrictors	Ergot alkaloids
Drugs that contain oestrogen	Oral contraceptives Oestrogen therapy
Drug withdrawal	Clonidine Opiates Cocaine
Drug interactions with antihypertensive drugs	Tricyclic antidepressants Indomethacin

Social history

The social history should include risk factors for hypertension and cardiovascular disease, such as high intake of alcohol, high consumption of salt and fat, lack of exercise, and smoking history. Some patients may report stressful lifestyles and domestic stress. Somewhat surprisingly, smoking is less common in patients with hypertension than the general population, but, when present, it greatly increases the risk of heart attack or stroke. The only exceptions are in patients with malignant hypertension and renal artery stenosis, which are closely associated with cigarette smoking.

Physical examination

Physical examination of patients with hypertension should assess the causes and seek evidence of target organ damage (for example, in the brain, heart, kidneys, and peripheral arteries). Cardiovascular risk factors and complications that may influence management should also be assessed. Height and weight should be measured so that body mass index (weight $(kg)/(height (m)^2)$) can be calculated to measure obesity. Body weight should be checked at every clinic visit.

Blood pressure should be measured as accurately as possible (see chapter 4). Current guidelines recommend that it is measured routinely in all adults at least every five years. It should be measured annually in patients with high-normal blood pressure (systolic 130–139 mm Hg; diastolic 85–89 mm Hg) and those with previously high readings that have settled. More frequent readings should also be taken in those with existing cardiovascular disease and/or diabetes mellitus.

General

Physical examination may show typical facies of systemic disease, such as thyroid disease, acromegaly, or Cushing's syndrome. Other clues include xanthomas or xanthelasmas (associated with hyperlipidaemia), nicotine staining of the fingers, and facial plethora, which may indicate polycythaemia or excessive intake of alcohol.

Cardiovascular

Examination of the pulse may show a full volume pulse and occasionally atrial fibrillation. Absent pulses or arterial bruits suggest atherosclerotic vascular disease in the femoral or carotid circulation. Such patients may have undiagnosed atheromatous renal artery stenosis, which will affect the choice of antihypertensive drug.

Examination of the praecordium may show cardiomegaly or left ventricular heave. Cardiac auscultation may show a loud second heart sound or heart murmurs, or both, which would merit further investigation. For example, aortic regurgitation results in a soft blowing early diastolic murmur, which is associated with a wide pulse pressure ("collapsing pulse") and isolated systolic hypertension.

One rare vascular cause of hypertension is suggested by the presence of a loud systolic murmur across the chest and back, with delayed femoral pulses and a difference in blood pressure recorded in the arms and legs as a result of coarctation of the aorta. The femoral pulses should be checked for radiofemoral delay in all patients with newly diagnosed hypertension.

Chest

Examination of the chest may suggest obstructive airway disease (such as asthma, chronic bronchitis, or emphysema) that would mean that β blockers should not be used. Fine basal crackles suggest pulmonary oedema or fibrosing alveolitis.

History

History	Comment
Angina, myocardial infarction, or stroke	• Complications of hypertension • Angina may improve when blood pressure is controlled, especially with β blockers
Asthma, obstructive airways disease, and heart failure	• Preclude the use of β blockers • Angiotensin converting enzyme inhibitors indicated in patients with heart failure
Diabetes	• Angiotensin converting enzyme inhibitors preferred
Polyuria or nocturia	• Suggests renal impairment
Claudication	• May be aggravated by β blockers • Atheromatous renal artery stenosis may be present
Gout	• May be caused by diuretics
Arthritis	• Some non-steroid anti-inflammatory drugs increase blood pressure
Family history of hypertension	• Important risk factor
Family history of premature death	• May have been the result of hypertension
Family history of diabetes	• Patient also may be diabetic
Cigarette smoker	• Independently causes coronary heart disease and stroke
High alcohol intake	• A cause of high blood pressure
High salt intake	• Important to advise restriction of salt
Stressful lifestyle	• Usually not relevant in long term

Single one-off raised blood pressure readings can be misleading. Regular measurement of blood pressure gives a truer picture of a patient's blood pressure over time. Ambulatory blood pressure measured over 24 hours is useful in some patients

Blood pressure measurement

- Use properly maintained, calibrated, and validated device
- Routinely measure blood pressure when patient is sitting; blood pressure when patient is standing should be recorded at the initial examination in elderly patients or those with diabetes
- Remove tight clothing, support upper arm at heart level, ensure hand relaxed, and avoid talking
- Use cuff of appropriate size
- Take at least three readings; more readings needed if marked differences between initial measurements
- Do not treat on basis of isolated high reading
- Routinely check blood pressure is same in both arms at first visit; if no difference is found, use nearest arm only in future examinations
- With mercury sphygmomanometer only:
  —Lower mercury column slowly (2 mm per second)
  —Read blood pressure to the nearest mm Hg
  —Measure diastolic blood pressure as disappearance of sounds (phase V)

Examination

Finding	Comment
Retinal haemorrhages and exudates with or without papilloedema	Malignant hypertension Patient should be admitted
Plethoric appearance	Consider Cushing's syndrome or high intake of alcohol
Obesity	Body mass index >25 kg/m^2
Intermittent sweating, anxiety, pallor, or weight loss	Consider phaeochromocytoma
Myxoedema or thyrotoxicosis	Give rise to hypertension
Tachycardia	Consider anxiety but exclude thyrotoxicosis
Left ventricular apical heave	Left ventricular hypertrophy is an ominous sign Urgent treatment needed
Loud aortic second sound	Present in patients with long-established hypertension
Mitral incompetence murmur	May be the result of left ventricular failure
Aortic outflow murmur	May be a flow murmur, but aortic stenosis may be present May be aortic sclerosis if second sound loud
Pulmonary fine crepitations	Suggests heart failure Use diuretics first Consider angiotensin converting enzyme inhibitors
Pulmonary wheezes	Avoid β blockers
Delayed or weak femoral pulses with precordial murmurs	Consider coarctation of the aorta Measure blood pressure in legs
Absent foot pulses	Arteriosclerosis
Abdominal mass	Autosomal dominant polycystic kidney disease or aortic aneurysm if pulsatile
Corneal arcus or xanthelasmae	Associated with hyperlipidaemia

Abdomen

Examination of the abdomen may provide additional clues to associates of hypertension. For example, a renal arterial bruit is suspicious of renal artery stenosis. Almost 50% of patients with severe hypertension and peripheral artery disease have evidence of renal artery stenosis on renal angiography. Occasionally, such patients present with flash pulmonary oedema. Stigmata of chronic liver disease may be present as a result of high intake of alcohol. Polycystic kidneys may also be palpable on abdominal examination.

Central nervous system

Examination of the central nervous system may show cerebrovascular disease. Cognitive function is rarely tested in hypertension clinics, but informal assessment may show impairment in patients with vascular dementia.

Fundus

Fundoscopy should be part of the initial clinical assessment of all patients with severe hypertension. Patients with severe hypertension and retinal haemorrhages, cotton wool spots, hard exudates, with or without papilloedema are diagnosed as having malignant hypertension. Without treatment, 90% of patients with this condition die within two years. These patients need immediate hospital referral. Many have renal impairment or heart failure, although some present clinically with only visual symptoms.

If the blood pressure is <200/110 mm Hg, routine examination of the optic fundi is not particularly helpful, as retinopathy of grades 1–2 on the Keith, Wagner, and Barker scales is more closely related to age and generalised cardiovascular status than the level of the blood pressure. Diabetic retinopathy and the changes that result from hypertension may be difficult to assess. Fundal photography through dilated pupils should be performed if retinopathy is present or suspected.

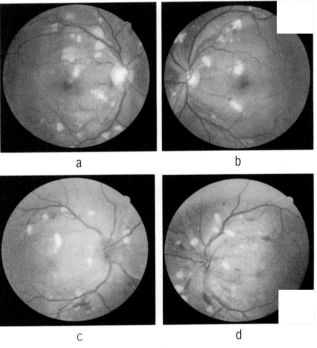

a   b

c   d

Retinal features in two patients with malignant phase hypertension: grade III (top) and grade IV retinopathy (bottom). Reproduced from Lip GY, et al. *J Human Hypertens* 1997;11:395–6

7 Investigation in patients with hypertension

G Y H Lip, D G Beevers

Routine investigations

Investigations are needed in all patients with hypertension to detect any underlying cause (for example, to exclude secondary hypertension), assess for the consequences of hypertension (target organ damage), and test for other cardiovascular risk factors. Thorough investigations should be performed in young patients (those younger than 40 years), patients who present with severe or resistant hypertension, and patients in whom secondary hypertension is suspected. Chest x ray, urine microscopy and culture, and echocardiography are not "routine" investigations but may be needed in some patients.

Urinalysis

Proteinuria and microscopic haematuria suggest intrinsic renal disease, including glomerulonephritis (particularly immunoglobulin A nephropathy), polycystic kidney disease, or pyelonephritis. In patients with proteinuria, the risk of mortality and morbidity is roughly doubled for a given blood pressure.

Biochemistry

Serum levels of potassium

Serum levels of potassium are usually low or low-normal in patients with primary hyperaldosteronism (Conn's syndrome). This is often associated with high or high-normal serum levels of sodium.

Low levels of potassium sometimes occur in patients who take diuretics, but if hypokalaemia is marked, doctors should check for another underlying cause of hypertension (such as primary aldosterone excess or Conn's syndrome). Patients with malignant hypertension may have mild hypokalaemia because of aldosterone excess, which is secondary to high levels of renin caused by juxtaglomerular cell ischaemia. As blood pressure is brought under control, this hypokalaemia often normalises. If serum levels of potassium remain low without diuretic treatment despite good control of blood pressure over a few months, primary hyperaldosteronism should be excluded.

Hyperkalaemia may develop in patients with renal failure and those who take drugs such as angiotensin converting enzyme inhibitors, angiotensin receptor blockers, and potassium sparing diuretics (for example, spironolactone and amiloride). Spironolactone is increasingly used as third line treatment in patients with resistant hypertension, and potassium and renal function need to be monitored regularly. Low salt alternatives, which contain potassium salts, should be used cautiously with angiotensin converting enzyme inhibitors as dangerous hyperkalaemia can occur.

Levels of sodium in serum

Serum levels of sodium may be high or high-normal in patients with primary hyperaldosteronism (Conn's syndrome). This is usually associated with low serum levels of potassium. In patients with secondary hyperaldosteronism as a result of malignant hypertension or renal disease, serum levels of sodium can be low or low-normal. Low levels of sodium may also be present with overuse of diuretics. Profound hyponatraemia, which may cause confusion and hypotension, is occasionally seen in patients on low doses of diuretics.

Serum levels of urea and creatinine

Non-malignant essential hypertension only rarely causes renal impairment, but associated comorbid disease (such as diabetes)

Routine investigations in all patients

- Blood pressure measurement and possibly ambulatory blood pressure measurement
- Urine dipstick test for protein and blood
- Serum creatinine and electrolytes
- Blood glucose (ideally after fasting)
- Levels of total and high density lipoprotein cholesterol in serum (ideally after fasting)
- Electrocardiography

Proteinuria and haematuria

- Dipstick proteinuria and haematuria may occur in patients with:
  — Primary renal disease
  — Non-malignant hypertension (hypertensive nephrosclerosis)
  — Renal arteriolar fibrinoid necrosis as a result of malignant hypertension
- Dipstick proteinuria should be investigated further by quantification of protein excretion over 24 hours
- Haematuria can occur in patients with:
  — Malignant and non-malignant hypertension
  — Urological disease
- Dipstick glycosuria suggestive of coincident diabetes mellitus

---

First line investigations

Investigation	Comments
Urine testing:	
Proteinuria	• Hypertensive damage, diabetic nephropathy, or intrinsic renal disease
Haematuria	• Common in patients with hypertension • Glomerulonephritis should be excluded • Consider cytoscopy
Glycosuria	• Suggests diabetes mellitus
Biochemistry:	
Sodium	• High (145–155 mmol/l) in primary hyperaldosteronism
Potassium	• Low (1.5–3.4 mmol/l) as a result of diuretic treatment and in chronic renal disease and primary hyperaldosteronism
Creatinine	• High in hypertensive renal damage or intrinsic renal disease • Better test than urea
Calcium	• High in primary hyperparathyroidism, which is associated with hypertension
Aspartate or γ glutamyl transpeptidase	• High in patients who consume excess alcohol with or without liver disease
Uric acid	• High in hypertension, patients who take diuretics, and heavy drinkers
Total cholesterol and high density lipoprotein	• Must be measured in all patients with hypertension to calculate cardiovascular risk
Non-fasting blood glucose	• Screening for diabetes
Haematology:	
Haemoglobulin	• High in some cases of essential hypertension and patients with excessive intake of alcohol • Low in chronic renal failure
Mean cell volume	• High in patients with high alcohol intake
Low platelet count	• Consider connective tissue disease
Electrocardiogram	• Chest lead criteria for left ventricular hypertrophy: R wave in V5 + S wave in V1 $\geq$35 mm. ST depression in lead V5 or V6 indicates left ventricular "strain"
Chest x ray	• Not reliable for left ventricular hypertrophy • Only if patient is breathless • Rib notching in coarctation of aorta

and concomitant treatment (such as angiotensin converting enzyme inhibitors or angiotensin receptor blockers) can lead to renal impairment.

Intrinsic renal disease can cause hypertension, and levels of urea and creatinine in serum should be part of the initial work up in a patient with newly diagnosed hypertension. Even a modest increase in levels of creatinine in serum needs more detailed investigation.

Levels of creatinine thus need to be monitored regularly, especially if renal impairment is initially present. A reciprocal serum creatinine chart (that is, a plot of the reciprocal of levels of creatinine in serum against time) is useful to indicate the rate of deterioration of renal function and the need for nephrological assessment. It is a big jump to dialysis!

Other parameters

High levels of uric acid in serum are found in about 40% of patients with hypertension, especially in association with renal impairment. Increased ingestion of alcohol and the use of thiazide diuretics can also lead to higher levels of uric acid. Whether high levels of uric acid are harmful in their own right or only by association with hypertension remains uncertain.

Abnormal results of liver function tests may be found in association with excessive intake of alcohol. The main non-specific abnormality is an increase in levels of γ glutamyl transferase, often in association with macrocytosis. A close association exists between abuse of alcohol and hypertension.

High levels of liver enzymes are also seen in patients with non-alcoholic hepatic steatosis (fatty liver). This is found in association with hypertension and type 2 diabetes, particularly in those who are overweight as part of the metabolic syndrome.

A low serum level of calcium with a high level of phosphate may be found in patients with renal failure. Hypertension is closely associated with primary hyperparathyroidism, which results in a high level of calcium and a low serum level of phosphate. Serum levels of calcium are also slightly higher in patients who use thiazide diuretics.

Lipids

Assessment of serum levels of lipids is mandatory—as part of the assessment of cardiovascular risk. In outpatient clinics, a simple random level of serum cholesterol together with high density lipoprotein cholesterol will suffice. The ratio of total cholesterol to high density lipoprotein cholesterol can therefore be calculated.

Haematology

A full blood count is not needed in most patients with hypertension. Macrocytosis may suggest associated alcohol abuse or hypothyroidism, while polycythaemia may be primary (polycythaemia ruba vera—a rare cause of hypertension), stress related (Gaisbok's syndrome), or secondary to causes such as renal carcinoma or, more commonly, obstructive airways disease or high intake of alcohol.

Electrocardiography

12 Lead electrocardiography is a mandatory part of the assessment of patients with hypertension. It provides a baseline with which later changes may be compared, but, more importantly, it may show evidence of the presence of left ventricular hypertrophy—the most common manifestation of hypertensive target organ damage. Left ventricular hypertrophy is diagnosed most often when the sum of the S wave in lead V1 and the R wave in leads V5 and V6 is ≥35 mm (Sokolow-Lyon criteria). The prognosis is even worse if the "strain" pattern with ST shift and T inversion is also seen in leads V5 or V6, or both. In very

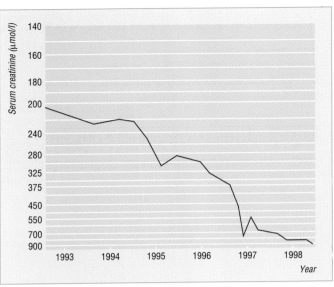

Reciprocal creatinine chart in a patient with chronic renal failure. Adapted from Beevers DG, MacGregor GA. *Hypertension in practice.* London: Martin Dunitz, 1999

> To quantitate total cardiovascular disease risk, it is necessary to measure serum total and high density lipoprotein (HDL) cholesterol levels

> In patients with abnormal lipid levels, more detailed assessment, including measurement of fasting serum levels of lipids (including triglycerides), is needed

> Almost all patients with hypertension and diabetes need statin drugs if they are at high cardiovascular risk—even if their lipid profiles are not abnormal

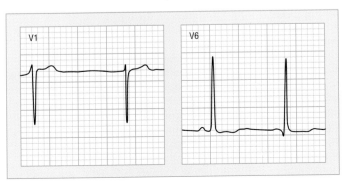

Electrocardiogram showing left ventricular hypertrophy and strain

obese patients, these chest criteria may be negative due to the thick chest wall. Left ventricular hypertrophy should be suspected if there is left axis deviation and/or a tall R wave in lead aVL.

In addition, 12 lead electrocardiography may show underlying ischaemic heart disease, including previous myocardial infarction. Common arrhythmias, such as atrial fibrillation, may also be documented.

Investigations for selected patients

If clinical assessment or the initial simple investigations suggest the need for further detailed investigation, specialist advice may be needed to facilitate management and further tests.

Echocardiography
Left ventricular hypertrophy may be seen in echocardiograms in patients with severe hypertension in whom electrocardiograms show no evidence of hypertrophy. Echocardiography should be performed in patients with breathlessness to assess cardiac function. Hypertension can lead to heart failure as a result of systolic dysfunction alone or secondary to associated myocardial infarction, when regional abnormalities of wall motion may be present. In patients with hypertension who develop atrial fibrillation, assessment of left atrial size and valves, as well as ventricular size and function, may influence decisions on cardioversion and antithrombotic treatment.

Echocardiography may also show impaired diastolic function with reduced diastolic filling but normal contractive (systolic) function. The significance of left ventricular diastolic dysfunction is uncertain.

Twenty four hour urine collection
At least one urine collection over 24 hours should be taken to test for urine catecholamines in young, thin patients with hypertension and those with paroxysmal symptoms, including blanching attacks, panic attacks, and marked variability of blood pressure. Routine estimation of creatinine clearance is not necessary unless the serum creatinine is raised. Estimates often are inaccurate because of inadequate urine collection. Creatinine clearance can be estimated with the Cockroft and Galt formula.

Measurement of sodium excretion in urine over 24 hours may give some indication of the intake of salt and provide a basis for education and counselling. If dipstick urinalysis shows proteinuria, 24 hour collection of urine allows this to be quantified. If the patient has > 1 g proteinuria per 24 hours, referral to a nephrologist may be needed for consideration of renal biopsy.

Radiology and imaging
Chest radiography
Chest x rays are not helpful in most patients with hypertension—unless they are breathless. Rib notching may be seen in patients with coarctation of the aorta.

Renal imaging
Renal ultrasound is the best imaging test for suspected renal disease and should be performed in all patients with malignant hypertension, proteinuria, or raised serum levels of creatinine. All patients younger than 40 years with hypertension and those with severe or resistant hypertension should also undergo renal ultrasound scans. A unilateral small kidney raises the suspicion of renal artery stenosis, although unilateral renal parenchymal disease cannot be ruled out. In patients with some forms of glomerulonephritis, the kidney may seem "bright" or echogenic

Other electrocardiographic features of hypertension
- Left axis deviation
- Tall R wave in lead aVL (> 12 mm)
- Deep S wave in lead V1
- Tall R wave in leads V5 or V6
- Biphasic P wave in leads V4-V6
- ST-T inversion leads V4-V6 (strain)

Paradoxically, echocardiography should be considered if electrocardiograms (ECGs) unexpectedly are normal. An ECG is an insensitive method of detecting left ventricular hypertrophy, particularly in obese patients

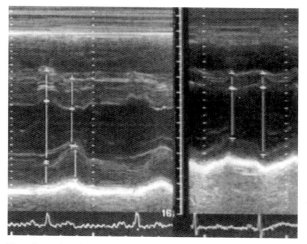

Two dimensional and M mode echocardiograms showing severe left ventricular hypertrophy with marked thickening of the intraventricular septum and posterior wall (left) and normal echocardiogram (right)

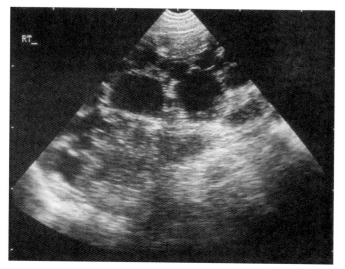

Ultrasound showing polycystic kidney

on ultrasound images. More often, chronic renal parenchymal disease, in which the renal cortex is thinned or the renal pelvis is distorted and dilated, or both, can be diagnosed. Hydronephrosis or polycystic kidneys can also be diagnosed. Improvements in renal ultrasound techniques mean that intravenous urography is no longer used.

Magnetic resonance renal angiography is the most useful test for renal artery stenosis. If this is positive, conventional renal angiography may be needed for more detailed assessment of the renal arteries. Renal artery stenosis may be the result of atheroma in elderly patients and fibromuscular dysplasia in young patients (particularly women).

Computed tomography and magnetic resonance imaging
Computed tomography and magnetic resonance imaging are the investigations of choice for detecting phaeochromocytomas and adrenal tumours that cause cortisol or aldosterone excess. These tests may miss small tumours in patients with Conn's syndrome and may not pick up generalised adrenal hyperplasia.

Radioisotope imaging
Renal radioisotope imaging has a limited role in the investigation of hypertension. The captopril renogram was previously used for the diagnosis of renal artery stenosis but has been superceded by magnetic resonance renal angiography.

Plasma levels of hormones
Plasma levels of hormones must be assessed in patients with suspected endocrine causes of hypertension. Many of these hormones are labile and the blood must be taken carefully with special blood tubes—often with the patient fasting and supine and preferably before they rise in the morning. Such tests are performed best in specialist centres.

Conn's syndrome is diagnosed by high plasma levels of aldosterone and suppressed plasma renin activity. More recently, the aldosterone-renin ratio has been used to detect aldosterone excess at an earlier stage, when absolute levels of hormone are equivocal. Secondary hyperaldosteronism causes high plasma levels of aldosterone in association with high plasma renin activity. This is seen in some patients with renal or renal artery disease and those who use diuretics.

Cushing's syndrome is investigated by the overnight dexamethasone suppression test. Acromegaly is suspected from the typical facies and is investigated with a glucose tolerance test and plasma levels of growth hormone. A skull x ray may show an enlarged pituitary fossa, which can be confirmed on computed tomographs.

Primary hyperparathyroidism is suspected biochemically because of the presence of a normal or high level of parathyroid hormone in the presence of high serum levels of calcium. Tumours can be localised by ultrasound or computed tomography, or both.

In patients with phaeochromocytoma, secretion of adrenaline, noradrenaline, and dopamine may be intermittent. These hormones or their metabolites (metanephrines) thus are usually measured in a collection of urine over 24 hours. This test should be done in young, thin patients with hypertension who have variable hypertension, tachycardia, blanching attacks, or other episodic symptoms.

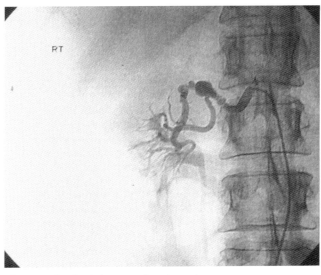
Fibromuscular dysplasia on renal angiography

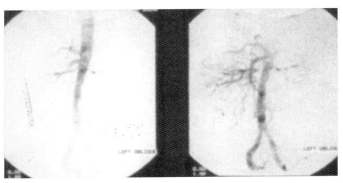
Renal angiograms showing atheromatous renal artery stenosis (left) and extensive aortic atheroma (right)

Overnight dexamethasone suppression test to detect Cushing's syndrome
- Patient takes 1 mg of dexamethasone at 22:00
- The next morning, the patient's plasma level of dexamethasone should be < 50 mol/l
- Failure to suppress suggests Cushing's disease or Cushing's syndrome

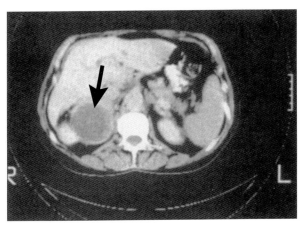
Computed tomograph of phaeochromocytoma

8 Non-pharmacological treatment of hypertension

G Y H Lip, D G Beevers

Many lifestyle factors increase blood pressure, and their modification can reduce blood pressure in patients with or without hypertension. Changes that lead to such reductions include restriction of salt intake, weight reduction, reduced intake of dairy products, increased intake of fruit and vegetables, moderation of alcohol intake, and increased exercise. These approaches may reduce the need for drug treatment, add to or complement the effect of antihypertensive drugs, and even occasionally allow antihypertensive drugs to be stopped. Effective non-pharmacological lifestyle modification may reduce blood pressure as much as a single antihypertensive drug. Combinations of two or more lifestyle modifications produce even better results.

In patients with mild hypertension but no cardiovascular complications or target organ damage, the response to non-pharmacological measures should be observed for 4–6 months. If antihypertensive drugs are introduced—for example, in patients with more severe hypertension—non-pharmacological lifestyle measures should be started concurrently. The fourth guidelines of the British Hypertension Society also recommend that verbal and written advice on lifestyle measures be given to all patients with hypertension and those with high-normal blood pressure or a strong family history of hypertension.

These non-pharmacological approaches should also be applied in a population based strategy to manage blood pressure in the community. Such a strategy could theoretically minimise the increase in blood pressure with age and thus reduce the prevalence of hypertension, as well as the burden of cardiovascular disease to the community.

Obesity and weight reduction

Obesity and hypertension are closely related, and some people have an additional link with insulin resistance and diabetes mellitus. Every attempt should therefore be made to encourage obese patients with hypertension to start and maintain a weight reducing diet. The input of dieticians to this strategy is crucial and allows patients to achieve more weight loss than the advice of medical staff alone.

In general, reductions in systolic and diastolic blood pressures occur with weight loss. For example, a weight loss of 3 kg results in an average decrease in blood pressure of 7/4 mm Hg; a weight loss of 12 kg results in a decrease of 21/13 mm Hg.

Weight reduction also has beneficial effects on risk factors associated with hypertension, such as insulin resistance, diabetes, dyslipidaemia, and left ventricular hypertrophy. The blood pressure reducing effect of weight reduction should be complemented by an increase in physical exercise and a reduction in the intake of salt and alcohol.

Salt intake and salt restriction

Many studies confirm a clear and causal relation between dietary intake of salt and blood pressure. Conversely, a strategy of salt restriction to <100 mmol/day (<6 g/day) significantly reduces blood pressure. A reduction in salt intake from an average of 10 g/day (about two teaspoons) to 5 g/day can result in an average reduction in blood pressure of 5/2 mm Hg.

Reductions in salt intake can result in larger decreases in blood

---

British Hypertension Society guidelines: lifestyle modifications for primary prevention and treatment of hypertension

- Maintain normal body weight for adults (body mass index 20–25 kg/m²)
- Reduce dietary sodium intake to <100 mmol/day (<6 g/day sodium chloride or <2.4 g/day sodium)
- Engage in regular aerobic physical activity, such as brisk walking (≥30 minutes per day on most days of the week)
- Limit alcohol consumption to ≤3 units/day in men and ≤2 units/day in women
- Consume a diet rich in fruit and vegetables (for example, at least five portions a day)
- Consume a diet with low levels of saturated and total fat

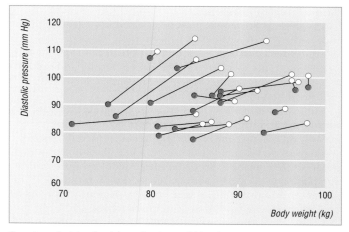

Overview of trials of weight reduction and blood pressure change. Adapted from Staessen J, et al. *J Human Hypertens* 1988;2:207–17

Potential benefits of weight loss of 10 kg in patient who weighs 100 kg

Variable	Effect
Blood pressure	• Decrease in systolic blood pressure and diastolic blood pressure of 10 mm Hg
Diabetes mellitus	• 50% lower risk of developing diabetes • 30–50% decrease in fasting levels of blood glucose • 15% decrease in haemoglobin subtype A1c • 30–40% decrease in deaths related to diabetes
Plasma lipids	• 10% decrease in levels of total cholesterol • 15% decrease in levels of low density lipoprotein cholesterol • 30% decrease in levels of triglycerides • 8% increase in levels of high density lipoprotein cholesterol

Adapted from Royal College of Physicians.

pressure in the elderly, African-Caribbean people (who are more salt sensitive), and those with higher initial blood pressures. On average, one third of such patients who reduce their intake of salt will achieve a reduction in blood pressure of 5/5 mm Hg.

The effects of salt restriction add to the beneficial effects of a healthy diet in reducing blood pressure. For example, in the dietary approaches to stop hypertension (DASH) trial, salt restriction further lowered blood pressure in patients who had already obtained benefit from a diet low in dairy products and rich in fruit and vegetables.

Salt restriction can be achieved by not adding salt at the dining table or when cooking and by reducing intake of salty foods, such as crisps, hamburgers, sausages, and salty bacon. A large amount of salt also is present in common everyday processed foods, such as bread, breakfast cereals, "ready meals," and flavour enhancers, such as stock cubes.

Substitution by salt substitutes (which contain potassium salts instead of sodium salts) is another option, but care is needed when angiotensin inhibitors or potassium sparing diuretics are used, as hyperkalaemia may result.

Alcohol

High intake of alcohol can be related to hypertension, as well as obesity and other problems, including cardiac arrhythmias, alcoholic cardiomyopathy, neuropathy, liver disease, and pancreatitis. In patients with hypertension, even a moderately high intake of alcohol of 80 g/day (equivalent to four pints of beer a day) can significantly increase blood pressure. Binge drinking has been associated with an increased risk of stroke.

Conversely, reducing intake of alcohol to fewer than 21 units a week reverses any increase in blood pressure associated with alcohol, and blood pressure remains low in those who continue to abstain. Patients with hypertension should therefore be advised to limit their alcohol intake to fewer than 21 units a week in men and 14 units a week in women.

Exercise and physical activity

Epidemiological studies on exercise and blood pressure are often confounded by "healthy lifestyle" changes, including changes in diet and weight reduction. It generally is accepted, however, that a graduated exercise programme beneficially can reduce mean blood pressure in patients with hypertension. Such physical activity should be regular and aerobic (such as brisk walking) and, importantly, should be tailored to each patient. For example, three vigorous training sessions a week may be appropriate for fit younger patients, and brisk walking for 20 minutes a day may be more appropriate in older patients. Such regular aerobic exercise reduces systolic and diastolic blood pressures by about 2–3 mm Hg, but a combination of exercise and a healthy diet may reduce systolic and diastolic blood pressures by 5–6 mm Hg. A reasonable strategy is perhaps one that includes regular aerobic exercise (such as brisk walking) for at least 30 minutes, ideally on most, but at least three, days of the week.

In contrast, isometric exercise (such as heavy weight lifting) is not recommended because of the pressor effects on blood pressure. Obese patients with newly diagnosed hypertension and heart disease should not suddenly take up heavy exercise, although a sensibly administered physical exercise programme may be beneficial.

In observational studies, physical activity—at work or in leisure time—is associated with a lower risk of coronary heart disease in men and women. This cardioprotection is lost when exercise is discontinued. The greatest reduction in risk is seen

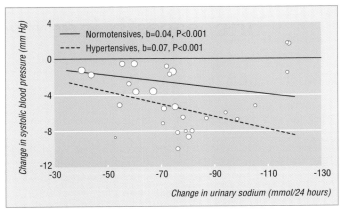

Dose response of salt restriction: meta-analysis of trials ≥1 month longer. A 6 g/day reduction in intake of salt predicts a fall in systolic blood pressure of 7 mm Hg in hypertensives and 4 mm Hg in normotensives. Adapted from He FJ, MacGregor GA. *J Human Hypertens* 2002;16:761–70

> **One slice of bread contains 0.5 g of salt**

> **Evidence from population studies show that modest alcohol consumption up to the recommended limit (especially with red wine—the French paradox) has some protective effect against coronary heart disease**

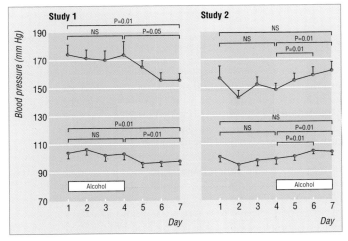

Restriction of alcohol in hypertension. (NS = not significant.) Adapted from Potter JF, Beevers DG. *Lancet* 1984;i:119–22

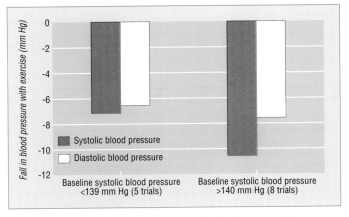

Exercise and blood pressure: meta-analysis of trials. From Arrol B, Beaglehole R. *J Clin Epidemiol* 1992;45:439–47

between sedentary and moderately active individuals; the difference between those who take moderate and vigorous activity is more modest.

Healthy diet

The dietary approaches to stop hypertension (DASH) trial clearly shows a beneficial effect on blood pressure of a diet high in fruit and vegetables and low in dairy products. Increased consumption of fruit and vegetables has a beneficial effect on blood pressure. An increase from two to seven portions of fruit and vegetables a day reduces average blood pressure by about 7/3 mm Hg in patients with hypertension. Increased fruit and vegetable consumption and decreased consumption of dairy products and total and saturated fats can cause larger reductions—perhaps 11/6 mm Hg—in patients with hypertension. This beneficial effect may be partly the result of increased intake of potassium.

Total dietary intake of fat should be reduced to ≤35% of total energy intake. Intake of saturated fats should be limited to one third of the total intake of fats; saturated fats can be replaced by an increased intake of monounsaturated fats. In clinical practice, such diets reduce serum levels of cholesterol by only about 6% on average.

Increases in dietary intake of potassium through increased consumption of fruits and vegetables may reduce blood pressure. The use of potassium tablets to supplement intake of potassium is not recommended, however, especially if angiotensin converting enzyme inhibitors or potassium sparing diuretics are used.

Other lifestyle interventions

Approaches to reduce stress can result in short term reductions in office blood pressure, but they have little effect on ambulatory blood pressure over 24 hours (that is, the more usual blood pressure). Only limited evidence supports the use of garlic, herbal, and other complementary medicines as strategies to reduce blood pressure.

Chronic and heavy cigarette smoking may be associated with hypertension. Indeed, blood pressure can increase acutely during smoking. Importantly, smoking has a graded adverse effect on cardiovascular risk, increasing it even more than mild hypertension. People who stop smoking rapidly reduce their risk by as much as 50% after one year, although 10 years may be needed before the level of risk reaches that of people who have never smoked.

Patients with hypertension who smoke should therefore be encouraged to stop smoking. Interventions with doctor's advice and encouragement can reduce smoking by 21%, which will be reinforced by smoking cessation clinics. Nicotine replacements can help smoking cessation and are generally safe in people with hypertension.

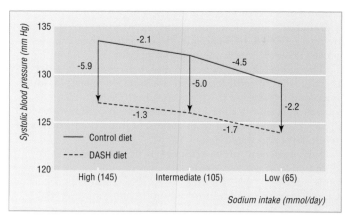

DASH trial: diet and salt restriction. Adapted from Sacks FM, et al. *N Engl Med* J 2001;344:3–10

The beneficial effects of fish oils on blood pressure and cardiovascular disease remain uncertain. Hooper L, et al (*BMJ* 2006;332:752–60) have questioned the available trial data

---

Evidence does not support the use of calcium, magnesium, or potassium supplements alone or in combination

---

PREMIER trial (a randomised trial to determine the effects of multi-component lifestyle interventions on blood pressure)

- Randomised trial recently tested multicomponent lifestyle interventions on blood pressure in demographic and clinical subgroups
- Participants randomised to groups that received:
  —Advice only
  —Established recommendations
  —Established recommendations plus the diet of the dietary approaches to stop hypertension (DASH) trial (see Elmer PJ, et al. *Ann Intern Med* 2006;144:485–95)
- Established recommendations plus diet:
  —Reduced blood pressure in patients of all ages and ethnic groups
  —Reduced blood pressure significantly more in older people

Approaches to reduce stress, some of which have produced small falls in office blood pressure

- Stress management
- Meditation
- Yoga
- Cognitive therapies
- Breathing exercises
- Biofeedback

9 Pharmacological treatment of hypertension

G Y H Lip, D G Beevers

When to use drugs

The commonly accepted definition of hypertension is "that level of blood pressure above which investigation and treatment do more good than harm." Reliable evidence now shows that patients whose blood pressure is consistently >160/90 mm Hg will obtain benefits from drugs that reduce blood pressure. Such treatment reduces the rate of stroke by about 40% and of heart attacks by about 20%. Thresholds are lower in high risk people, particularly those with diabetes and renal impairment.

Many patients with hypertension have poor control of blood pressure, many are not receiving any treatment, and inappropriate drugs are often initiated: low doses are started with no dose titration and unsuitable combinations are used. Two (or more) drugs that synergistically reduce blood pressure are better than high dose monotherapy, which has a higher risk of side effects. Randomised clinical trials consistently show that most patients with hypertension need two or more drugs to achieve targets for blood pressure.

Until recently, no single class of antihypertensive drugs was considered any more effective than another for reducing blood pressure. The losartan intervention for endpoint (LIFE) trial and Anglo-Scandinavian cardiac outcomes trial (ASCOT), however, strongly suggest that drug regimens based on β blockers with or without thiazide diuretics are less effective than more modern drugs at preventing strokes. Furthermore, β blockers were not superior to other drugs at preventing coronary heart disease.

Monotherapies reduce blood pressure by an average of 7–8%, with some interindividual variation. This is largely a reflection of individual pathophysiological mechanisms, with low renin states in elderly people, Afro-Caribbeans, and those with type 2 diabetes.

Thresholds

The British Hypertension Society's guidelines (2004) recommend that blood pressure should be measured on four separate occasions. If levels remain high, antihypertensive drugs should be prescribed on the basis of the results of 17 controlled trials of hypertension treatment. Decisions to start treatment in patients with mild hypertension are also made on the basis of careful history taking, including family history of premature heart attack or stroke, 12 lead electrocardiography, and levels of total and high density lipoprotein cholesterol. Decisions also are influenced by the patient's attitude to taking drugs for life, their motivation, and their awareness of the risks of hypertension and the benefits of treatment.

The European guidelines, the guidelines of the World Health Organization and International Society of Hypertension, the guidelines of the American Joint National Committee (JNC VII), and the National Institute for Clinical Excellence's guidelines are broadly similar to the British Hypertension Society's. All stress the assessment of total cardiovascular risk, with thresholds depending on risk rather than blood pressure. Guideline committees all stress that patients whose blood pressures are near to these thresholds or settle to below them need particular care with regular monitoring (1–2 times a year).

Decisions on treatment for patients at lower levels of cardiovascular risk will be influenced by the patient's attitude to treatment and the benefit anticipated from treatment. Blood pressure will increase within five years to levels that clearly need treatment in about 10–15% of such patients. In addition,

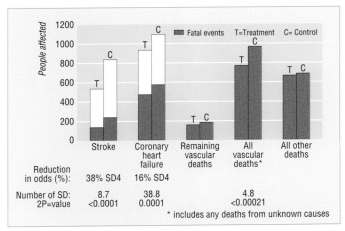

Meta-analysis of the benefits of blood pressure lowering in 17 randomised controlled trials

Two recent long term outcome trials (LIFE (losartan intervention for endpoint) and ASCOT-BPLA (blood pressure lowering arm of the Anglo-Scandinavian cardiac outcomes trial)) have shown that β blockers are less effective than other drugs at preventing strokes. The latest British Heart Society guidelines (BHS 4) now suggest that β blockers should be used only in patients with coronary heart disease

British Society of Hypertension's thresholds for starting antihypertensive treatment

- All patients whose blood pressures persistently exceed 160 mm Hg systolic or 100 mm Hg diastolic, or both
- Patients with systolic pressures of 140–159 mm Hg or diastolic pressures of 90–99 mm Hg, or both, if they have target organ damage, type 2 diabetes, or a total risk of cardiovascular disease ≥20% at 10 years

Note: Decisions on treatment must be based on total cardiovascular risk and not just coronary risk, as strokes now outnumber heart attacks in patients with hypertension

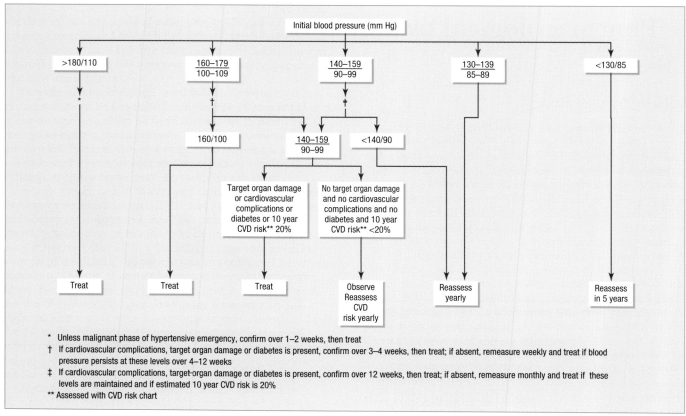

Blood pressure thresholds and drug treatment in hypertension

cardiovascular risk will increase with age, so risk should be reassessed annually. All of these patients should be encouraged to continue with lifestyle measures to reduce blood pressure and cardiovascular risk.

Targets

Treatment should be optimised to achieve optimal blood pressure targets. These targets are often difficult to achieve or may be achieved only at the expense of a major reduction in quality of life. The British Hypertension Society's guidelines thus also recommend ideal targets and audit targets that must be achieved if possible.

Optimal blood pressure targets
- <140/85 mm Hg in low risk patients
- <130/80 mm Hg in high risk patients

Antihypertensive drugs

Diuretics
Thiazide diuretics and thiazide like diuretics
Thiazide diuretics (such as bendroflumethiazide) and the thiazide like diuretics (chlorthalidone and indapamide) are cheap, easy to use, and can be given once daily. They are effective and are the drugs of choice in elderly people and those of African origin. They are also useful in combination with angiotensin converting enzyme inhibitors, angiotensin receptor blockers, and β blockers.

The thiazides reduce blood pressure by increasing excretion of sodium and water, which lowers blood volume, but they also have some vasodilating properties. The reduction in blood volume results in reflex activation of the renin-angiotensin-aldosterone system, which leads to an increase in peripheral vascular resistance that may attenuate the reduction of blood pressure. This effect is smaller in patients with low

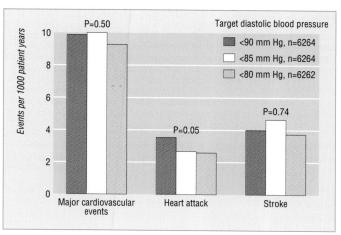

Main results from the hypertension optimal treatment (HOT) trial

baseline plasma levels of renin (such as in elderly people and those of African origin).

The antihypertensive effect of thiazides is slow, and the dose-response curve is relatively flat, so that increasing doses give limited additional reductions in blood pressure. The adverse metabolic effects of the thiazides are increased at higher doses, however, which exacerbates hypokalaemia, hyperuricaemia, and hyperglycaemia. The lowest possible doses are therefore used—for example, bendrofluazide 2.5 mg once a day.

Marked hypokalaemia is very uncommon with the use of thiazides in low doses. If hypokalaemia occurs, therefore, other causes must be considered, particularly underlying aldosterone excess (such as occurs in patients with Conn's syndrome).

Impairment of glucose tolerance and development of overt type 2 diabetes are more common when thiazides (particularly in high doses) are combined with β blockers. Minor changes in plasma levels of lipids and uric acid may also be seen; these are of limited clinical importance if low doses are used.

Loop diuretics
Loop diuretics (such as frusemide) are less potent at reducing blood pressure than the thiazides. They should be used only when a patient has concomitant cardiac or renal failure.

Potassium sparing diuretics
The potassium sparing diuretics—spironolactone, amiloride, and triamterene—control sodium and potassium exchange in the distal renal tubes. They limit the loss of potassium in patients treated with other diuretics, although no convincing evidence shows that they add to the antihypertensive effects.

In patients with "resistant" hypertension who are already receiving an angiotensin blocking drug, the addition of spironolactone in low doses can produce impressive reductions in blood pressure. Significant increases in serum levels of potassium may occur, so careful monitoring is mandatory. Spironolactone is also used in the treatment of patients with aldosterone excess and the preoperative management of patients with Conn's syndrome. Spironolactone and a new selective aldosterone receptor blocker, eplerenone, used in combination with angiotensin converting enzyme inhibitors reduce mortality and morbidity in patients with left ventricular impairment as a result of myocardial ischaemia. Limited information is available on the use of eplerenone in patients with hypertension.

Side effects include hyperkalaemia and renal impairment, so monitoring of renal function is important. The non-selective aldosterone antagonist, spironolactone, may have antiandrogen effects, causing gynaecomastia and sexual dysfunction in men. This side effect appears not to occur with the use of eplerenone.

β Blockers
Most β blockers reduce cardiac output through negative chronotropic and inotropic effects. The short term haemodynamic responses are partly offset by reflex activation of vasoconstrictor mechanisms, which may attenuate reductions in blood pressure. Release of renin from the kidneys is also partly blocked. As with the thiazide diuretics, the β blockers have a relatively flat dose-response curve for reductions in blood pressure. As their mechanism of action involves suppression of renin, they tend to be less effective than monotherapy in elderly people and African-Caribbeans, although this can be overcome with concomitant use of diuretics.

The fourth guidelines of the British Hypertension Society recommend β blockers only in patients with specific indications, such as heart disease. Carvedilol, bisoprolol, and metoprolol are beneficial in patients with heart failure as a result of left ventricular systolic impairment. β Blockers are indicated in patients after myocardial infarction, in those with angina, and

Activation of the renin-angiotensin-aldosterone system can be reduced with the concomitant use of drugs that block this system, particularly the angiotensin converting enzyme inhibitors and angiotensin receptor blockers. This explains why there is useful synergy of diuretics with drugs that block the renin-angiotensin-aldosterone system

Erectile dysfunction develops in up to 25% of men who take thiazide diuretics in higher doses, although this may be less of a problem with indapamide

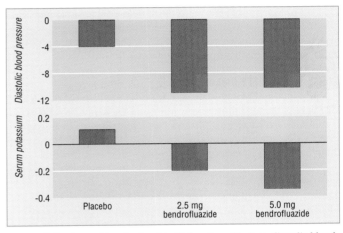

Effects of placebo and bendrofluazide (2.5 or 5 mg/day) on diastolic blood pressure and serum levels of potassium

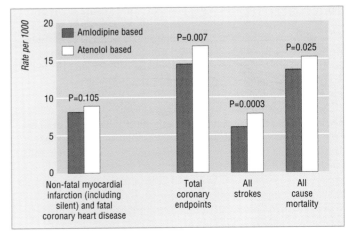

Results of the blood pressure lowering arm of the Anglo-Scandinavian cardiac outcomes trial (ASCOT-BPLA)

in some patients with atrial fibrillation. Otherwise, the β blockers should rarely be used in the management of asymptomatic and uncomplicated hypertension

Recent evidence from clinical trials suggests that β blockers may increase the likelihood of new onset diabetes, especially when combined with thiazide diuretics. In patients with electrocardiographically confirmed left ventricular hypertrophy, the β blocker atenolol was less effective than the angiotensin receptor blocker losartan in reducing stroke. In addition, the blood pressure lowering arm of the Anglo-Scandinavian cardiac outcomes trial was stopped early because of the inferiority of treatment based on a thiazide and the β blocker atenolol compared with treatment based on amlodipine and perindopril.

Side effects of β blockers include lethargy, aching limbs on exercise, impaired concentration and memory, erectile dysfunction, vivid dreams, sleep disturbance, and exacerbation of symptoms of peripheral artery disease and Raynaud's syndrome. β Blockers are contraindicated absolutely in patients with bronchospasm or heart block. They may cause minor adverse metabolic effects, including impairment of blood glucose tolerance and lipid abnormalities (such as reduced levels of high density lipoprotein cholesterol and high levels of triglycerides), although the clinical significance is likely to be limited. They should not be used in conjunction with verapamil.

The newer β blockers, carvedilol, nebivolol and bisoprolol, have not been tested in long-term outcome trials in hypertension. Whether they share the inferiority of the older β blockers in hypertension is therefore unknown.

Calcium channel blockers

Calcium channel blockers act by inhibiting the transfer of calcium ions across smooth muscle cell membranes, which produces arteriolar vasodilatation. The systolic hypertension in Europe (SYST-EUR) trial and two other long term outcome trials validated their use as first line drugs in patients with hypertension.

Calcium channel blockers are useful antianginal and antihypertensive drugs. Non-dihydropyridine calcium channel blockers (diltiazem and verapamil) block calcium channels in cardiac myocytes. This reduces cardiac output and may have some antiarrhythmic action on the atrioventricular node.

The dihydropyridine calcium channel blockers (such as nifedipine, amlodipine, and felodipine) block L type calcium channels in vascular smooth muscle cells. This causes vasodilatation and reductions in vascular resistance and arterial blood pressures. These agents have little effect on the atrioventricular node but do have some mild diuretic effects.

Some formulations of dihydropyridine calcium channel blockers (such as short acting nifedipine capsules) have a rapid onset of action and unpredictable effects on blood pressure, and they may cause reflex sympathetic stimulation, tachycardia, and activation of the renin-angiotensin-aldosterone system. Nifedipine capsules bitten or swallowed should never be used in the treatment of hypertensive emergencies and urgencies. Longer acting formulations of dihydropyridine calcium channel blockers (such as nifedipine LA, amlodipine, and felodipine) cause less neurohumoral activation.

Side effects include headache and flushing, but the most troublesome side effect is dose dependent peripheral oedema. This is the result of transudation of fluid from the vascular compartments into the dependent tissues because of precapillary arteriolar dilatation. It is not responsive to diuretics. Gum hypertrophy is common with dihydropyridine calcium channel blockers but is seen rarely with verapamil or diltiazem. Non-dihydropyridine calcium channel blockers cause less peripheral oedema, but they are negatively inotropic and negatively chronotropic.

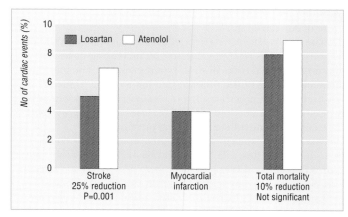

Losartan v atenolol in patients with hypertension and electrocardiographically confirmed left ventricular hypertrophy in the losartan intervention for endpoint (LIFE) study

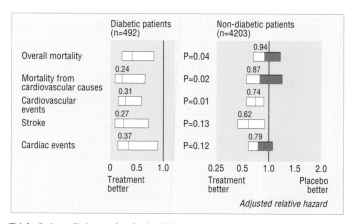

Trial of nitrendipine v placebo in diabetic and non-diabetic elderly patients with isolated systolic hypertension in the systolic hypertension in Europe (SYST-EUR) trial

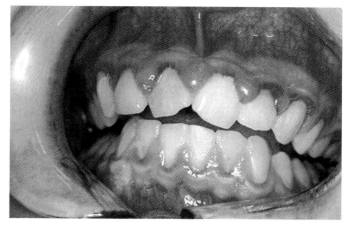

Gum hypertrophy caused by amlodipine

All calcium channel blockers, but particularly verapamil, can alter bowel habit and occasionally cause troublesome constipation. This side effect can be turned to a benefit in some patients with irritable bowel syndrome and hypertension

Angiotensin converting enzyme inhibitors

The angiotensin converting enzyme inhibitors are a major class of drugs that has transformed the treatment of cardiovascular disease. As the name implies, these drugs block angiotensin converting enzyme, which converts angiotensin I to angiotensin II, mainly in the lungs. Angiotensin II is a potent vasoconstrictor and also stimulates aldosterone release from the adrenal cortex, which causes retention of sodium and water. The angiotensin converting enzyme inhibitors thus cause vasodilatation and, to a lesser extent, reduced renal absorption of sodium and water. In addition, angiotensin II has many other properties that may be harmful in vascular disease, and its inhibition (at the local tissue and systemic levels) leads to additional benefits. Angiotensin converting enzyme is also responsible for the breakdown of bradykinin, and angiotensin converting enzyme inhibitors increase levels of bradykinin, which enhances vasodilatation.

In patients who are fluid depleted, usually because of high doses of diuretics, and those with severe heart failure, bilateral renal artery stenosis, and malignant phase hypertension, acute administration of angiotensin converting enzyme inhibitors may cause a sudden decrease in blood pressure and deterioration in renal function, so caution is needed. Increases in serum levels of creatinine <20% are the result of reversible reductions in intraglomerular pressure, however, and are acceptable. In the long term, angiotensin converting enzyme inhibitors preserve renal function and are indicated in most patients with hypertension and renal impairment.

The most common side effect of angiotensin converting enzyme inhibitors is a persistent dry cough, which occurs in 10–20% of users. It is most common in women who do not smoke, although the complaint sometimes comes from the patient's partner. These drugs can cause life threatening acute or subacute angio-oedema, with swelling of the tongue and lips. This occurs in about one in 4000 white patients but is four times more common in black people.

Angiotensin receptor blockers

The angiotensin receptor blockers block type I angiotensin II receptors (AT_1), which leads to vasodilatation and reductions in blood pressure. They are a relatively new class of drugs, but clinical experience is growing and is impressive. Like the angiotensin converting enzyme inhibitors, these drugs are not only excellent drugs for hypertension but have benefits in stroke reduction, heart failure with left ventricular dysfunction, nephropathy (diabetic and non-diabetic), and after myocardial infarction, where they are at least as good as the angiotensin converting enzyme inhibitors.

In relation to long term outcomes in hypertension, the angiotensin receptor blockers are superior to β blockers. In the losartan intervention for endpoint (LIFE) study, losartan was superior to atenolol in reducing strokes and fewer cases of new onset diabetes were diagnosed. In the valsartan antihypertensive long-term use evaluation (VALUE) trial, a regimen based on valsartan was not superior to a regimen based on amlodipine, although valsartan was associated with fewer cases of new onset diabetes.

α Blockers

The α blockers block the activation of alpha-1 adrenoceptors in the vascular tree, which results in vasodilatation. Prazosin, the early α blocker, was short acting and had to be given three times a day, so it is no longer recommended. Longer acting agents, such as doxazosin and terazosin, are now available. The doxazosin arm in the antihypertensive and lipid lowering treatment to prevent heart attack trial (ALLHAT) was terminated early, however, because of the suggestion of more adverse outcomes with α blockers than thiazide diuretics—principally a 25% excess

> Angiotensin converting enzyme inhibitors are not only excellent drugs for hypertension but also have benefits in patients after myocardial infarction, stable coronary artery disease, stroke, heart failure with left ventricular dysfunction, diabetic retinopathy, and diabetic and non-diabetic nephropathy

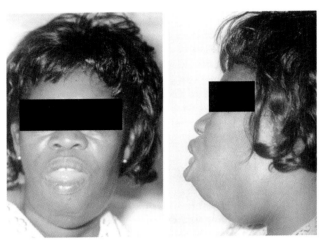

Acute angio-oedema caused by enalapril in an African-Caribbean patient

> Current knowledge means that angiotensin converting enzyme inhibitors and angiotensin receptor blockers are contraindicated absolutely in pregnancy and should be avoided in women who are likely to become pregnant

> As angiotensin receptor blockers are selective for the AT_1 receptors, they do not potentiate bradykinin, so cough and acute angio-oedema are very rare, and these agents are generally tolerated very well

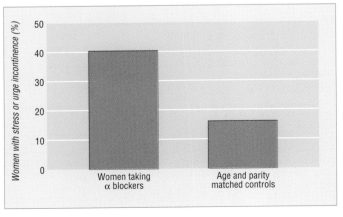

α Blockers and urinary incontinence in women

in alleged heart failure. α Blockers thus are considered to be third or fourth line drugs for hypertension and should be used with caution in patients at risk of heart failure.

Postural hypotension is a problem, especially with prazosin. All members of this drug class often cause stress or urge incontinence in women, who may not volunteer this adverse effect unless asked. By contrast, α blockers may be useful in men with prostatism. Minor benefits on levels of lipids and coagulation factors have not translated into clinically significant benefits.

> Alpha blockers have only been tested in one long-term outcome trial (ALLHAT). In this study, doxazocin was inferior to a diuretic as first line therapy. Alpha blockers can only therefore be justified as a last resort as third or fourth line drugs in resistant hypertension

Centrally acting agents

Methyldopa, clonidine, and moxonidine are centrally acting imidazoline agonists. Their central α agonism is thought to be responsible for their side effects: tiredness, lethargy, and depression. Almost no long term data are available on these drugs, which can therefore be justified only as a last resort in patients with resistant hypertension.

> Methyldopa can be used in pregnant women with hypertension, in whom long term follow-up shows that this agent is safe, with no adverse effects on the fetus, otherwise this agent has no place in the treatment of hypertension

Direct acting vasodilators

The main drugs in this class are hydralazine and minoxidil. Hydralazine is rarely used in hypertension, but it is of benefit when used in conjunction with nitrates in patients of African origin who have heart failure. Minoxidil, used with a diuretic and a β blocker, is occasionally needed in the treatment of severe resistant hypertension. The main side effect is hair growth, which almost precludes its use in women. It also causes tachycardia and fluid retention.

Choice of antihypertensive drugs

Each major class of antihypertensive drug has compelling indications and contraindications in specific patient groups. When no special considerations apply, the choice of initial antihypertensive drug should follow the ACD algorithm described on page 53.

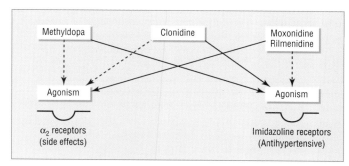

Central antihypertensive agents (selective imidazoline receptor agonists)

British Hypertension Society's indications and contraindications for the major classes of antihypertensive drugs

Class of drug	Indication		Contraindication	
	Compelling	Possible	Possible	Compelling
α Blockers	Prostatism	Dyslipidaemia	Postural hypotension	Urinary incontinence
Angiotensin converting enzyme inhibitors	Heart failure Left ventricular failure Type I diabetic nephropathy	Chronic renal disease* Type II diabetic nephropathy	Renal impairment* Peripheral vascular disease†	Pregnancy
Angiotensin II receptor antagonists	Cough induced by angiotensin converting enzyme inhibitors‡	Heart failure Intolerance of other hypertensive drugs	Peripheral vascular disease†	Pregnancy Renovascular disease
β Blockers	Myocardial infarction Angina	Heart failure§	Heart failure**	Asthma Chronic obstructive pulmonary disease Heart block
Calcium antagonists (dihydropyridine)	Isolated systolic hypertension in elderly patients	Angina Elderly patients	–	–
Calcium antagonists (rate limiting)	Angina	Myocardial infarction	Combination with β blockade	Heart block Heart failure
Thiazides	Elderly patients	–	Dyslipidaemia	Gout

*Angiotensin converting enzyme inhibitors may be beneficial in patients with chronic renal failure but should be used with caution. Close supervision and specialist advice are needed when patients have established and significant renal impairment.
†Angiotensin converting enzyme inhibitors and angiotensin II receptor antagonists should be used with caution in patients with peripheral vascular disease because of an association with renovascular disease.
‡If angiotensin converting enzyme inhibitor indicated.
**β blockers may worsen heart failure, but they may be used by specialists to treat heart failure.

First line drugs

The choice of first line antihypertensive drugs depends on the presence or absence of other important underlying medical conditions related to hypertension, pre-existing cardiovascular damage due to the hypertension, or other unrelated conditions. Finally the choice is greatly influenced by the patient's age and ethnicity—both of which affect release of renin.

Despite these factors, the prime objective is to control the blood pressure by any means. The differences in outcome between the different drug classes are minor compared with the differences attributable to the adequate control of blood pressure. In order to achieve good control of blood pressure, most patients need two or more antihypertensive drugs, so the choice of second and third line agent will also be influenced by the considerations above.

Several systems or algorithms have been devised to help doctors decide which drugs to use first and which to add in. All are in broad agreement, so this chapter concentrates on the British Hypertension Society's ACD system and the Birmingham hypertension square.

Second line drugs

Significant synergy of action occurs when an angiotensin blocking drug or β blocker is added to a thiazide diuretic or calcium channel blocker. Conversely, little synergy occurs when a calcium blocker is added to a diuretic or an angiotensin blocker is added to a β blocker. This is the rationale for the ACD system and the Birmingham hypertension square but with increasing disinclination to use the β blockers unless they are indicated specifically. At this stage, therefore, the regimen should be "A plus C or D" or "C or D plus A." Some doubt exists over whether much is gained from using an angiotensin converting enzyme inhibitor with an angiotensin receptor blocker, except possibly in patients with diabetic or non-diabetic nephropathy.

Third line drugs

The British Hypertension Society and Birmingham hypertension square agree that the next step is A + C + D.

Fourth line drugs

The guidelines provide little help with choice of fourth line drug, and doctors should apply strategies for patients with resistant hypertension. If a fourth drug is really indicated, several possibilities exist:

- In women, add spironolactone 25–50 mg once a day
- In men, add doxazosin 4–8 mg once a day
- Consider adding in a β blocker
- Try adding moxonidine 400 µg once a day
- Try adding minoxidil 5–10 mg three times a day.

Factors that affect first line choice of antihypertensive

Important underlying medical conditions related to hypertension	Pre-existing cardiovascular damage because of hypertension	Unrelated conditions
• Diabetes mellitus • Intrinsic renal disease	• Stroke • Heart attack • Heart failure	• Pregnancy • Obstructive airway disease • Bladder function

A(B)CD system

A—angiotensin blocking agents first

- Angiotensin converting enzyme inhibitors (if side effects are a problem, the angiotensin receptor blockers) are the drugs of first choice in:
    - Patients with stable heart failure
    - Patients with left ventricular dysfunction as result of myocardial ischaemia
    - Patients with most forms of primary renal disease
    - Patients with diabetic nephropathy
    - Possibly all patients with diabetes
    - Patients with a history of intolerance to other drug classes

B—β blockers first

- β Blockers should now be regarded as first line agents in only a minority of patients including:
    - Patients who have survived a heart attack
    - Patients with angina pectoris
    - Patients with stable heart failure
    - Patients with some tachycardias, including atrial fibrillation
- They may ameliorate some symptoms in hyperanxious patients

C—calcium blockers first

- Calcium blockers can be used as first line drugs:
    - In patients in whom thiazide diuretics are contraindicated or have caused clinical or metabolic side effects in the past
    - In men of African origin who are of sexually active age
- They may be beneficial in patients with peripheral vascular disease or Raynaud's phenomenon

D—diuretics first

- Thiazide diuretics used in low dose are the drugs of first choice in women and older patients with hypertension
- They have been well validated in long term outcome trials and are relatively free of side effects

Other drugs first

- Methyldopa is the drug of choice in pregnant women with hypertension
- The α blocker, doxazosin, occasionally may be the drug of choice in men with symptoms because of prostatic enlargement

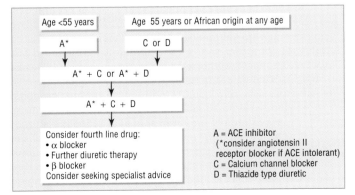

Treatment of newly diagnosed hypertension. β Blockers are not used except for patients with acute myocardial infarction/angina/congestive cardiac failure

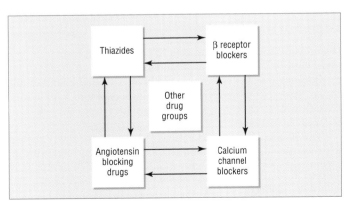

Birmingham hypertension square

Most patients will need two or more drugs to achieve treatment targets for blood pressure. This is true for complex cases in a hospital based context, as well as in primary care. The general approach is to use several drugs in low doses rather than one drug in high doses. This should minimise the side effects of drugs and give better control of blood pressure.

Strategies for resistant hypertension

Even with assiduous adherence to the recommendations above, a considerable number of patients in primary and secondary healthcare settings fail to reach ideal targets for blood pressure or even audit standards. In such patients, doctors should have a strategy for investigation and management. Many patients with resistant hypertension can be managed by adhering to the advice of the guideline committees. Many such patients, however, may benefit from referral to a specialist hypertension clinic for more detailed investigation and management.

Hypertensive urgencies and emergencies

Urgencies
Initially, malignant phase hypertension with retinopathy of grade III–IV is usually treated with 10–20 mg oral slow release nifedipine. Amlodipine, which has a gradual onset of action, is not suitable. Blood pressure should be monitored every 15 minutes. Sublingual nifedipine capsules bitten or swallowed should never be used, as the antihypertensive effect is unpredictable and often excessive. Atenolol has also been used successfully in hypertensive urgencies, but it is suitable only if no suggestion of phaeochromocytoma exists. Similarly, angiotensin converting enzyme inhibitors and angiotensin receptor blockers are best avoided until suspected renal artery stenosis is excluded. Normalisation of blood pressure over a few days or weeks is best achieved with gradual titration of drug doses according to the British Hypertension Society's ACD system.

Emergencies
Blood pressure needs to be brought down within minutes in a very small number of patients. In such cases, intravenous infusions of labetolol or intramuscular hydralazine may be useful. Sodium nitroprusside by intravenous infusion can control blood pressure accurately but should only be used in an intensive care unit.

Patients with severe hypertension and acute myocardial infarction need emergency reduction of blood pressure, particularly if thrombolysis is proposed. Intravenous nitrates, nitroprusside, or labetolol are best used in the coronary care unit.

Lipid lowering

Hyperlipidaemia is often present in combination with hypertension (> 50% of cases) and greatly adds to the cardiovascular risk. Treatment should be with stringent dietetic advice. Statins (3-hydroxy-3-methylglutaryl coenzyme A inhibitors) are safe and effective drugs that substantially reduce the risk of coronary heart disease and stroke in patients at such high risk.

The British Hypertension Society's guidelines (2004) abolish the concept of a baseline cholesterol threshold for intervention with statins and reduce the threshold of cardiovascular risk at 10 years for the initiation of statins for primary prevention to ≥ 20%. Suggestions that antihypertensive drugs should be selected on the basis of their effects on serum levels of lipids are

---

Strategy for investigation and management of patients with resistant hypertension
- Is the patient actually taking the tablets prescribed?
- Does the patient understand the consequences of uncontrolled hypertension?
- Does the patient understand the proven value of reducing blood pressure?
- Has the patient received advice on lifestyle and dietary manoeuvres that can help reduce pressures?
- Is the patient complying with this advice?
- Does the patient really have resistant hypertension or is the blood pressure only high in the presence of doctors and nurses (the white coat effect)?
- Has the patient had ambulatory blood pressure measurement to exclude this possibility?
- Does the patient have an undiagnosed underlying renal or adrenal cause for the high blood pressure?
- Does the patient's tablet regimen comply with the ACD system recommended by the British Hypertension Society?

Hypertensive emergencies in which blood pressure must be reduced within minutes with parenteral antihypertensive drugs occur. Rapid reductions in blood pressure can be dangerous and can cause stroke, myocardial infarction, and acute prerenal renal failure

---

Conditions in which blood pressure needs to be reduced rapidly
- Very severe hypertension
- Dissecting aortic aneurysm
- Severe left ventricular failure due to hypertension
- Severe pre-eclampsia
- Eclampsia
- Hypertensive encephalopathy

Nifedipine should never be used in patients with recent myocardial infarction because of its proarrhythmic effect

---

Lipid lowering studies

Lipid lowering arm of Anglo-Scandinavian cardiac outcomes trial (ASCOT-LLA)
- Statin therapy with 10 mg/day atorvastatin reduced the risk of coronary heart disease and stroke in people with treated hypertension, even when blood pressure was controlled optimally
- Benefit achieved in people with average total cholesterol of only 5.5 mmol/l
- Risk reductions in coronary heart disease events:
    —Unrelated to baseline cholesterol levels
    —Consistent across whole range of levels of serum cholesterol

Heart protection study (HPS)
- Patients with hypertension derived a similar benefit with 40 mg/day simvastatin
- Benefits were:
    —Unrelated to baseline levels of cholesterol
    —Consistent across whole range of levels of serum cholesterol

---

controversial. The adverse effects on lipid profiles of thiazide diuretics and β blockers may influence outcomes, and attenuate the beneficial effects of the use of statins.

The results of the lipid lowering arm of the Anglo-Scandinavian cardiac outcomes trial strongly suggest that all patients with hypertension and a total cardiovascular risk of $\geq 20\%$ at 10 years should receive a statin in addition to antihypertensive drugs, regardless of the serum cholesterol levels.

Aspirin

Despite the recognised increased prothrombotic state found in patients with uncomplicated hypertension, the use of antithrombotic drugs, particularly aspirin, is debatable. Consensus has nearly been reached that patients with hypertension who have coronary heart disease or have had a stroke or a transient ischaemic attack should be prescribed aspirin. In the hypertension optimal treatment trial, aspirin had no effect in the primary prevention of stroke and only a small effect on coronary prevention; however, an excess of major bleeding side effects was seen.

Despite the greatly increased risk in patients with uncontrollable hypertension, aspirin is best avoided because of the risk of cerebral haemorrhage. The British Hypertension Society's guidelines on use of aspirin recommend aspirin only if the blood pressure is controlled.

The figure showing the meta-analysis of the benefits of blood pressure lowering is adapted from Collins R, MacMahon S. *Br Med Bull* 1994; 50:272–90. The figure of blood pressure thresholds is adapted from Williams B, et al. *J Human Hypertens* 2004;18:139–85. The two figures of the results from the hypertension optimal treatment trial are adapted from Hansson L, et al. *Lancet* 1988;351:1755–62. The figure on effects of placebo and bendrofluazide is adapted from Carlson M, et al. *BMJ* 1990;300:975–8. The figures showing the results of the Anglo-Scandinavian cardiac outcomes trial are adapted from Dahlöf B, et al. *Lancet* 2005;366:895–906. Results of the losartan intervention for endpoint study are adapted from Dahlöf B, et al. *Lancet* 2002;359:995–1003. Results of the systolic hypertension in Europe trial are adapted from Tuomilehto J, et al. *N Engl J Med* 1999; 340:677–84. The table of indications and contraindications is adapted from British Hypertension Society. *J Human Hypertens* 1999;13:569–92. Photograph of acute angio-oedema published with permission of the patient. Figure on α blockers and urinary incontinence in women is adapted from Marshall HJ, Beevers G. *Br J Clin Pharm* 1996;42:507–9. The figure showing treatment of newly diagnosed hypertension is adapted from the joint British Hypertension Society/National Institute for Health and Clinical Excellence guidelines. Birmingham Square is adapted from Lip GY, et al. *J Human Hypertens* 1998;12:761–3.

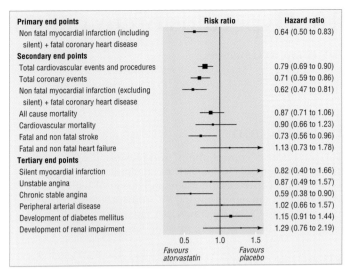

Lipid lowering arm of Anglo-Scandinavian cardiac outcomes trial (ASCOT-LLA)

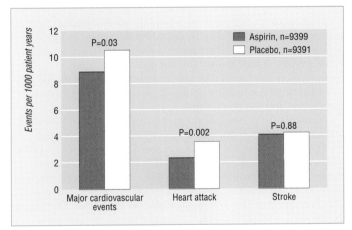

Results of the hypertension optimal treatment trial (HOT): aspirin substudy

10 Hypertension in patients with cardiovascular disease

G Y H Lip, D G Beevers

Introduction

The presence of "comorbidities" and previous cardiovascular diseases substantially influences the methods of assessing patients with hypertension, the management of high blood pressure, and the most appropriate antihypertensive drugs. As with all patients, total cardiovascular risk rather than just the height of the blood pressure must be taken into account.

Hypertension after stroke

As mentioned in chapter 1, hypertension is the most important treatable risk factor for stroke and antihypertensive treatment significantly reduces this risk. Half of all patients with stroke will have a history of hypertension, and up to 40% of patients are taking antihypertensive treatment when their stroke occurs.

Immediately after a stroke, a breakdown in cerebral autoregulation occurs. As a result, rapid decreases in blood pressure can cause a reduction in cerebral perfusion and a further extension of the stroke. For this reason, most authorities recommend that antihypertensive drugs should be withheld until the patient is ambulant; however, very little trial data is available on this point.

In the acute period after a stroke, casual levels of blood pressure are often high, with about 70% of patients having levels ≥140/90 mm Hg within the first 48 hours of ictus. These levels usually subside over the next 10–14 days. In part, the increase may be simply the result of the stress of hospitalisation, but other mechanisms may also be responsible, including pre-existing hypertension and neurohumeral activation. The higher the blood pressure at presentation, the worse the outcome, although patients who are hypotensive also do badly. The international stroke trial reported a J shaped relation between initial blood pressure and outcome, with early deaths increasing by 18% for every 10 mm Hg of admission systolic blood pressure below 150 mm Hg and by 4% for every 10 mm Hg above 150 mm Hg.

Some studies of β blockers and calcium blockers used immediately after a stroke have shown no benefit, but these studies were small. The recently reported acute candesartan cilexetil therapy in stroke survivors trial suggested that the angiotensin receptor blocker candesartan may be of benefit in patients with high blood pressure (200/110 mm Hg) within the first 48 hours after cerebral infarction. Whether existing antihypertensive drugs should be continued or stopped immediately after stroke is also unknown, and more trial data are awaited.

Treatment to reduce blood pressure in acute stroke (<48 hours) is probably appropriate when blood pressure is persistently very high (>220/110 mm Hg), although no robust outcome data from clinical trials are available on this point. In some countries, patients with acute cerebral infarction are given intravenous thrombolysis, but this is only feasible if computed tomography or magnetic resonance imaging of the head is available within two hours. If thrombolysis is given, then antihypertensive drugs—such as labetolol, nifedipine or intravenous sodium nitroprusside—will be needed. Immediate reductions in blood pressure may also be beneficial in patients

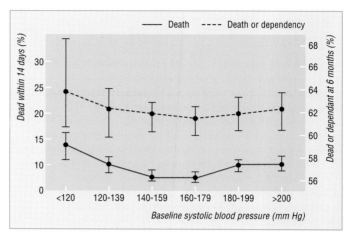

Blood pressure and clinical outcomes in 17 398 stroke patients in the International Stroke Trial

> **Low blood pressure may be related to an adverse prognosis in view of its association with large cerebral infarcts (total anterior cerebral artery occlusion) or concomitant cardiac disease**

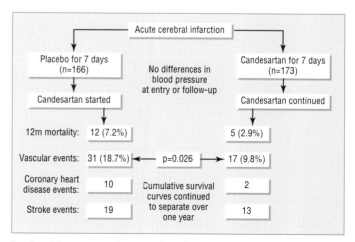

Results of the acute candesartan cilexetil therapy in stroke survivors (ACCESS) trial

with proven cerebral haemorrhage, aortic or carotid dissection, hypertensive encephalopathy, acute myocardial infarction, or angina. The situation in mild hypertension is less clear. No consensus exists on this issue and striking differences are seen in clinical practice between Europe and North America.

High blood pressures that persist for more than a month after a stroke are associated with an increased risk of recurrence, as well as the subsequent development of cardiovascular events. Data from seven randomised controlled intervention trials of reductions in blood pressure in patients with stroke or transient ischaemic attacks who were not necessarily hypertensive have shown that treatment significantly reduces the odds ratio for recurrence of fatal and non-fatal stroke by 26% and the odds ratio for cardiovascular events by 16%.

The perindopril protection against recurrent stroke study (PROGRESS) is the largest study to assess the effects of reductions in blood pressure (using the angiotensin converting enzyme inhibitor perindopril with or without the thiazide like diuretic indapamide) on recurrence in patients with a history of stroke or transient ischaemic attack with or without hypertension. This trial was confined to survivors of stroke seen in follow up clinics and provides no information on the management of acute stroke. A post hoc subgroup analysis of this trial suggested that the benefits of treatment were confined to patients who received perindopril with indapamine but not those who received perindopril alone. These findings, however, are controversial.

Patients who have had a transient ischaemic attack or cerebral infarct should receive aspirin (75–300 mg/day). This will reduce the risk of subsequent cardiovascular events by about 11% after acute stroke and by 20% in those with a past history of ischaemic stroke.

For patients with atrial fibrillation, anticoagulation will reduce the incidence of a further stroke by >65%, and treatment with statins reduces the risk of subsequent major vascular events by >20%. In patients with symptomatic severe carotid artery stenosis (≥70% but without near occlusion), carotid endarterectomy reduces subsequent stroke by 40%.

Left ventricular hypertrophy

Left ventricular hypertrophy is the most common cardiac manifestation of hypertensive end organ damage and is an independent risk factor for cardiovascular mortality. For a given level of blood pressure, the presence of left ventricular hypertrophy increases mortality by 3–4 times, and the risk is even greater if the patient has repolarisation abnormalities (the so-called strain pattern). Patients with left ventricular hypertrophy have a very high risk of stroke, myocardial infarction, heart failure, and atrial fibrillation.

Reliable evidence shows that drugs that block the renin-angiotensin-aldosterone system (angiotensin converting enzyme inhibitors and angiotensin receptor blockers) are better at reducing left ventricular hypertrophy than other drug classes. In the losartan intervention for endpoint (LIFE) study, for example, losartan caused more regression of left ventricular hypertrophy, which was reflected by 25% fewer strokes.

Electrocardiography is highly specific but not very sensitive for the detection of left ventricular hypertrophy—if an electrocardiogram shows left ventricular hypertrophy, it is usually present, but a normal electrocardiogram does not exclude left ventricular hypertrophy. The only exception is seen in slim adults, in whom chest leads may suggest left ventricular

Perindopril protection against recurrent stroke study (PROGRESS): perindopril or indapamide in survivors of stroke

Event	Active (n = 3051)	Placebo (n = 3054)	Per cent reduction (95% confidence interval)
Second stroke:	307	420	28 (17 to 38)
Ischaemic	246	319	24 (10 to 35)
Haemorrhagic	37	74	50 (26 to 67)
Acute myocardial infarction	115	154	26 (6 to 42)

Role of antihypertensives before, during, and after stroke

Before
Many randomised controlled trials have shown that aggressive treatment of hypertension is of benefit in patients with blood pressure > 140/85 mm Hg

During
Aggressive treatment of hypertension is detrimental to most patients. If the blood pressure is persistently > 180/110 mm Hg, prescribe 10–20 mg nifedipine or 25 mg atenolol. Previously prescribed antihypertensive drugs are best withdrawn and reinstated only at a later stage of the patient's recovery

After
On a long term basis, reduction of blood pressure prevents recurrence of stroke

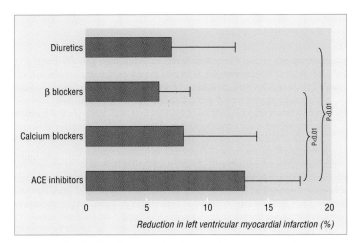

Overview of trials of antihypertensive drugs and regression of left ventricular hypertrophy (ACE inhibitors = angiotensin converting enzyme inhibitors)

hypertrophy that is not confirmed on echocardiography. Chapter 7 gives criteria for diagnosis of left ventricular hypertrophy.

Coronary heart disease

Patients with hypertension frequently have angina and myocardial infarction. Many antihypertensive drugs reduce blood pressure and have anti-ischaemic properties. In patients with hypertension, chest pain may result from impaired blood supply as a result of coronary artery atheromatous disease, but it can also result from "relative ischaemia," when significant left ventricular hypertrophy is present and is not accompanied by an increase in the coronary blood supply. Many patients with angina and hypertension have normal coronary arteries on angiography, and effective management of hypertension may improve the patient's symptoms.

All patients should receive aspirin (or clopidogrel, if aspirin is contraindicated) and a β blocker (unless contraindicated). One study showed some benefit from the use of the calcium antagonist verapamil after myocardial infarction if β blockers are contraindicated. Diltiazem may be beneficial after non-Q wave myocardial infarction with no evidence of heart failure or left ventricular dysfunction.

Dihydropyridine calcium blockers (especially short acting nifedipine) should be avoided, as evidence from trials shows these drugs can be harmful, possibly proarrhythmic, because of high plasma levels of catecholamines. Plasma potassium levels should be checked in patients who are taking thiazide diuretics for hypertension who are admitted with an acute myocardial infarction, because hypokalaemia leads to an increased tendency to arrhythmias and sudden death.

If patients with acute myocardial infarction have severe hypertension (>100/110 mm Hg), thrombolysis could be hazardous, with an increased risk of intracerebral bleeding. Before thrombolysis, therefore, blood pressure should be reduced with an oral β blocker, intravenous nitrates or, occasionally, sodium nitroprusside.

Angiotensin converting enzyme inhibitors are increasingly recognised to be of value in patients after myocardial infarction, especially if the patient has impaired left ventricular systolic function. Evidence shows that ramipril and perindopril reduce the rate of cardiovascular events even in patients with existing vascular disease.

Peripheral artery disease

A strong association exists between peripheral artery disease and hypertension, which is exacerbated by smoking. Although control of blood pressure is important in these patients, caution needs to be exercised with some drugs, particularly β blockers, which may occasionally worsen symptoms in patients with claudication. Nonetheless, data from trials do not suggest any worsening of the claudication distance in patients randomised to β blockers. Certainly, these drugs should not be used in patients with rest pain or gangrene.

Peripheral artery disease may increase the likelihood of undiagnosed atheromatous renal artery stenosis. Serum levels of creatinine should therefore be monitored carefully if angiotensin converting enzyme inhibitors are used. An increase in levels of creatinine ≤ 20% is acceptable, however, and not indicative of underlying atheromatous renal artery stenosis.

Hypertension in patients after a heart attack

- If the patient is receiving a thiazide diuretic, serum levels of potassium may be low, which means an increased risk of arrhythmias
- If blood pressure decreases, outcome is poor
- All patients should receive aspirin (or clopidogrel if aspirin is contraindicated)
- If blood pressure is very high, this must be reduced before thrombolysis is started
- All patients should receive a statin
- Dihydropyridine calcium blockers are contraindicated
- If possible, all patients should be given β blockers
- If β blockers are contraindicated, verapamil or diltiazem may be used
- Angiotensin converting enzyme inhibitors should be given if the patient has any evidence of left ventricular systolic dysfunction or clinical heart failure
- All treatments should be given, even if the blood pressure is not high

---

In the acute stages of myocardial infarction, blood pressure initially may be low. The diagnosis of hypertension could be missed and become apparent only at subsequent clinic visits or at attendance for cardiac rehabilitation

Angiotensin converting enzyme inhibitors may have anti-ischaemic, as well as antihypertensive, properties. They also reduce left ventricular after-load and reduce mortality in patients with heart failure due to left ventricular systolic dysfunction

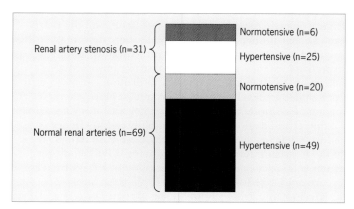

The prevalence of renal artery stenosis in patients with peripheral vascular disease

A recent Cochrane review on the treatment of patients with hypertension and peripheral arterial disease concluded that evidence for various antihypertensive drug classes in peripheral arterial disease was poor. Whether significant benefit or risk accrues from their use is therefore unknown. In view of this, definite recommendations on their use or avoidance cannot be given.

Patients with peripheral arterial disease need full cardiovascular risk assessment. They should be treated with antiplatelet drugs (aspirin or clopidogrel) and statins. Good control of hypertension and other associated disorders, such as angina, is needed.

Heart failure

At a population level, hypertension is commonly listed as an aetiological factor for the development of heart failure that results from systolic dysfunction. Patients with hypertension may develop heart failure because of underlying coronary artery disease or, occasionally, severe hypertension alone. Excessive alcohol intake could be a common aetiology for hypertension and alcoholic heart muscle disease—"alcoholic cardiomyopathy".

Heart failure with normal systolic function (so called "diastolic dysfunction" or "diastolic heart failure") is also commonly associated with hypertension and reflects impaired ventricular relaxation and poor cardiac compliance. Patients with diastolic heart failure tend to have a better prognosis than those with impaired systolic function (ejection fraction < 40%).

In the presence of heart failure as a result of systolic dysfunction, the use of verapamil is contraindicated and caution should be used with diltiazem. Treatment of systolic heart failure with diuretics and angiotensin converting enzyme inhibitors may control the patient's blood pressure. β Blockers (carvedilol, bisoprolol, or metoprolol) introduced slowly and gradually are beneficial—reducing mortality and morbidity.

The β blockers and angiotensin converting enzyme inhibitors have been proved to prolong life in patients with heart failure. They are therefore the drugs of choice for patients with systolic heart failure and hypertension. The use of carvedilol may have a small benefit over the use of metoprolol. The angiotensin receptor blockers are at least as good as the angiotensin converting enzyme inhibitors in patients with systolic heart failure and are a suitable alternative.

The aldosterone antagonist spironolactone has been shown to reduce mortality and morbidity in patients with heart failure. Great care must be taken when introducing this drug, particularly in patients with diabetes or renal impairment, as life threatening hyperkalaemia may develop. A new selective aldosterone antagonist eplerenone has been found to be beneficial in patients with heart failure after myocardial infarction. This drug has few of the adverse long term side effects of spironolactone (for example, gynaecomastia), but the results of trials with these drugs in patients with hypertension are awaited.

A smaller benefit in patients with heart failure is also seen with a combination of hydralazine and nitrates. This is not used often, unless angiotensin converting enzyme inhibitors and angiotensin receptor blockers are contraindicated or cause side effects. Hydralazine and nitrates may be the treatment choice in African-Caribbean patients with hypertension who develop heart failure, in whom angiotensin converting enzyme inhibitors may be less effective. A recent prospective randomised trial solely in African Americans (the African-American heart failure

> In the heart outcomes prevention evaluation (HOPE) study, many patients had peripheral arterial disease, and the use of ramipril resulted in a reduction in mortality and vascular morbidity compared with placebo

---

Antihypertensive drugs and peripheral vascular disease

- β blockers may worsen claudication
- Angiotensin converting enzyme inhibitors are hazardous if renal artery stenosis present
- Thiazides increase levels of lipids and glucose (small effect)
- Calcium channel blockers may relieve symptoms
- Lipid lowering drugs are often needed
- Type 2 diabetes mellitus is often present

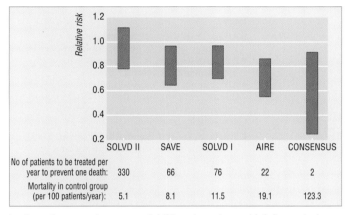

Angiotensin converting enzyme inhibitors in patients with left ventricular dysfunction. (AIRE = acute infarction ramipril efficacy; CONSENSUS = cooperative north Scandinavian enalpril survival study; SAVE = survival and ventricular enlargement; SOLVD = studies of left ventricular dysfunction)

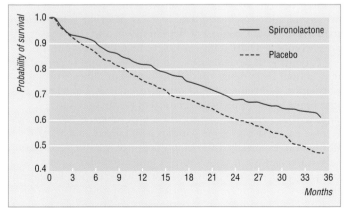

Survival curve for randomised aldactone evaluation study showing 30% reduction in all cause mortality when spironolactone (up to 25 mg) was added to conventional treatment in patients with severe chronic heart failure (New York Heart Association class IV)

trial) tested the effects of isosorbide dinitrate plus hydralazine on top of standard drugs in patients with New York Heart Association class 3–4 heart failure. It was stopped early after a significant survival benefit emerged among patients who received the additional treatment.

The best treatment for diastolic heart failure is less certain, but it includes treatment of concomitant hypertension and regression of left ventricular hypertrophy. Angiotensin converting enzyme inhibitors and β blockers (or rate limiting calcium antagonists) have been advocated. The candesartan in heart failure assessment of reduction in mortality and morbidity (CHARM)-preserved trial showed only a modest benefit of candesartan in patients with heart failure and normal systolic function.

Practical guidelines for antithrombotic treatment in patients with non-valvar atrial fibrillation

Assess risk and reassess regularly

Guideline	Risk of cerebrovascular accident		
	High*	Moderate†	Low‡
Type of patient	• All patients with previous transient ischaemic attack or cerebrovascular accident • All patients aged ≥75 years with diabetes, hypertension or vascular disease • All patients with clinical evidence of valve disease, heart failure, thyroid disease, and impaired left ventricular function on echocardiography**	• All patients aged <75 years with clinical risk factors: diabetes, hypertension, or vascular disease • All patients aged >65 years not in high risk group	• All patients aged <65 years with no history of embolism, hypertension, diabetes, or other clinical risk factors
Treatment	• Warfarin (target international normalized ratio 2–3) if no contraindications and possible in practice	• Warfarin (target international normalised ratio 2–3) or aspirin 75–300 mg/day • In view of insufficient clear cut evidence, treatment may be decided on individual cases • Referral and echocardiography may help	• Aspirin 75–300 mg/day

*Annual risk of cerebrovascular accident 8–12%.
†Annual risk of cerebrovascular accident 4%.
‡Annual risk 1%.
**Echocardiogram not needed for routine risk assessment but refines clinical risk stratification in case of moderate or severe left ventricular dysfunction and valve disease. A large atrium per se is not an independent risk factor on multivariate analysis.

Atrial fibrillation

Hypertension is a common aetiological factor for atrial fibrillation—the most common sustained disorder of cardiac rhythm. Both increase the risk of ischaemic stroke; when both are present, the risk is additive. The risk of stroke is higher in patients with poor control of hypertension, and those on antithrombotics have a higher risk of bleeding complications.

Patients with permanent atrial fibrillation and hypertension may benefit from drugs that allow control of the rate of fibrillation and reduce blood pressure, such as β blockers and rate limiting calcium channel blockers (verapamil and diltiazem), in addition to antithrombotic drugs. β Blockers may reduce paroxysms in some patients with paroxysmal atrial fibrillation, especially if the blood pressure is controlled. Some care is needed when class I and III antiarrhythmic agents are used in the presence of left ventricular hypertrophy, because of the risk of proarrhythmia. The risk of atrial fibrillation seems to be higher in patients with hypertension and hypokalaemia as a result of primary aldosteronism (Conn's syndrome).

Figure of blood pressure and clinical outcomes is adapted from Leonardi-Bee J, et al. *Stroke* 2002;33:1315–20. Acute Candesartan Cilexetil Therapy in Stroke Survivors trial is adapted from Schrader et al. *Stroke* 2003;34:1699–1703. Table of results from the perindopril protection against recurrent stroke study is adapted from PROGRESS Collaborative Group. *Lancet* 2001;358:1033–41. The figure of regression of left ventricular hypertrophy with antihypertensive drugs is adapted from Schmieder RE, et al. *JAMA* 1996; 275:1507–13. The figure of renal artery stenosis in peripheral vascular disease is adapted from Watchell M, et al. *J Human Hypertens* 1996;1:83–5. The figure showing angiotensin converting enzyme inhibitors in left ventricular dysfunction is adapted from Davey Smith G, Egger M. *BMJ* 1994;308:72–4. Survival curve for randomised aldactone evaluation study is adapted from Pitt B, et al. *N Engl J Med* 1999;341:709–17. The table showing practical guidelines for antithrombotic treatment in patients with non-valvar atrial fibrillation is adapted from Lip GYH, et al. *Lancet* 1999;353:4–6.

11 Special groups—diabetes, renal disease, and connective tissue disease

G Y H Lip, D G Beevers

Diabetes mellitus

Hypertension and type 1 and type 2 diabetes often coexist. Hypertension (≥140/90 mm Hg) is twice as common in people with diabetes than those without diabetes. For example, hypertension is very common (up to 80%) in patients with type 2 diabetes; in women, the increase in systolic blood pressure with age is also steeper. In patients with type 1 diabetes, the presence of hypertension is related strongly to incipient or overt diabetic nephropathy.

Furthermore, hypertension and diabetes are commonly associated with hyperlipidaemia. Hypertension therefore greatly increases the already high risk of coronary disease in people with diabetes—by twofold in men and fourfold in women. Patients with hypertension and diabetes also have double the risk of mortality of people with hypertension but not diabetes.

The aetiology of hypertension in patients with diabetes is multifactorial. In patients with type 1 diabetes, hypertension may be related to diabetic renal disease, as a result of marked activation of the renin-angiotensin-aldosterone system. Patients with type 2 diabetes may have volume expansion and sodium retention, perhaps related to hyperinsulinaemia. Plasma levels of renin and angiotensin tend to be low.

Reduction of blood pressure in patients with diabetes has marked benefits for major cardiovascular events, including heart failure, cardiovascular death, or total mortality. Cardiovascular risk is higher in patients with diabetes than those without at every level of blood pressure—even into the conventional "normotensive" range. Furthermore, no "threshold" below which risk substantially declines exists.

A decision to use antihypertensive treatment in patients with diabetes needs to take into account the effects of antihypertensive drugs on glucose and lipid metabolism. Furthermore, reductions in progression of retinopathy, microalbuminuria, albuminuria, and progression of nephropathy occur. For example, hypertension accelerates the decline of renal function in patients with diabetes and established nephropathy; conversely, treatment with antihypertensives slows the progression of nephropathy in patients with type 1 and type 2 diabetes. Some antihypertensive drugs may be better at preventing new onset diabetes: for example, in the losartan intervention for endpoint (LIFE) study, losartan was better in terms of this endpoint than atenolol.

Current guidelines recommend that reduction of blood pressure with drug treatments is indicated in people with type 1 or type 2 diabetes when the systolic blood pressure is ≥140 mm Hg or the diastolic blood pressure is ≥ 90 mm Hg. Targets for the treatment of blood pressure also are lower in patients with diabetes; the "optimal target" is <130/80 mm Hg.

Choice of therapy

Angiotensin converting enzyme inhibitors generally have been recommended as first line therapy for people with diabetes and hypertension because of their benefits on cardiac function, vascular disease, nephropathy, retinopathy, and possibly neuropathy. Nonetheless, in the antihypertensive and lipid lowering treatment to prevent heart attack trial (ALLHAT), which included more than 12 000 people with hypertension and type 2

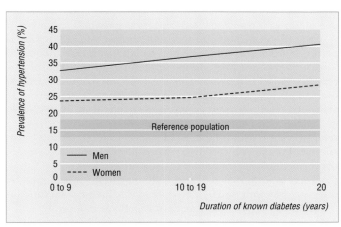

Hypertension in patients with diabetes

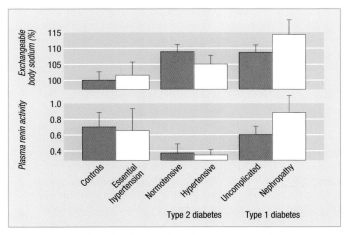

Levels of renin and total exchangeable sodium in patients with diabetes mellitus

---

Hypertension in patients with diabetes: key points from the British Hypertension Society's fourth guidelines

- Hypertension, especially systolic blood pressure, is more difficult to control to target in people with coexisting diabetes
- Most clinical trials have failed to achieve the recommended blood pressure targets, and reduction in systolic blood pressure to <140 mm Hg has been especially difficult
- Control of diastolic blood pressure is less problematic, but the main focus should be on control of systolic blood pressure; indeed, many patients (especially those with type 2 diabetes) have isolated systolic hypertension

---

diabetes, the angiotensin converting enzyme inhibitor lisinopril was not superior to thiazide diuretics or thiazide like diuretics in reducing coronary or cardiovascular events or mortality in people with type 2 diabetes.

The angiotensin receptor inhibitors are a suitable alternative to the angiotensin converting enzyme inhibitors and may have less troublesome drug side effects. The losartan intervention for endpoint (LIFE) study showed that treatment based on losartan was more effective than treatment based on atenolol at reducing cardiovascular events, cardiovascular death, and total mortality in patients with type 2 diabetes and hypertension.

Data also show the value of renoprotection with agents that act on the angiotensin-renin system in patients with type 2 diabetes. Angiotensin converting enzyme inhibitors and angiotensin receptor blockers delay progression from microalbuminuria to overt nephropathy and (for angiotensin receptor blockers, at least) progression of overt nephropathy to end stage renal disease.

Evidence in patients with type 1 diabetes shows renoprotection with inhibition of angiotensin converting enzyme, but data on cardiovascular protection with angiotensin converting enzyme inhibitors (or angiotensin receptor blockers) beyond that achieved with improved control of blood pressure is limited. Indeed, the rate of decline of renal function in patients with overt diabetic nephropathy is reduced by reductions in blood pressure and treatment with angiotensin converting enzyme inhibitors (or, as an alternative, angiotensin receptor blockers). Furthermore, progression from microalbuminuria to overt nephropathy is delayed. Whether the benefit of angiotensin converting enzyme inhibitors or angiotensin receptor blockers accrues from blockade of the renin-angiotensin system per se or the associated reduction in blood pressure, however, is unclear.

Most patients with hypertension and diabetes will need a combination of antihypertensive drugs (often three or more) to reach targets for blood pressure. The combination should include an angiotensin converting enzyme inhibitor or angiotensin receptor blocker. Low doses of thiazide diuretics or thiazide like diuretics, calcium blockers, and α blockers all are possible add on drugs. Some combined drugs can be prescribed as a fixed dose combination to improve drug compliance and reduce the costs of drugs.

Many people with type 2 diabetes and hypertension also benefit from treatment with statins—irrespective of baseline levels of cholesterol. In patients with type 1 diabetes, insufficient data with regard to statins are available, but the high rates of cardiovascular disease in this population mean they should be treated as for patients with type 2 diabetes.

The British Hypertension Society's guidelines also suggest low doses of aspirin for primary prevention of cardiovascular disease—but only when blood pressure is <150/90 mm Hg and the risk of cardiovascular disease at 10 years is >20%. Glycaemic control should be optimised, and non-pharmacological lifestyle measures, such as weight reduction, increased exercise, and restriction of dietary intake of sodium, should be implemented.

Renal disease

The frequency of renal impairment is higher in patients with hypertension—as a cause or effect of the high blood pressure. Renal parenchymal disease is the cause of hypertension in about 5% of people. Renal impairment itself is now recognised to be a powerful risk factor for cardiovascular disease, and some patients have an enormously increased chance of developing stroke, heart failure, or coronary heart disease.

The presence of high serum levels of creatinine or proteinuria at the initial assessment of a patient with

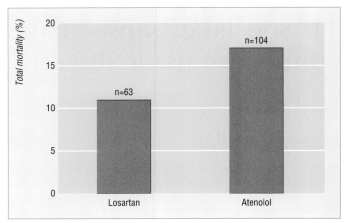

Diabetic substudy of the losartan intervention for endpoint (LIFE) study

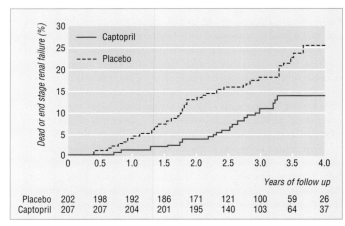

Angiotensin converting enzyme inhibitors in patients with type 1 diabetes

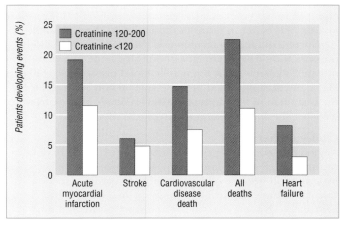

Renal impairment as a risk factor for cardiovascular disease

hypertension should lead to suspicion of renal parenchymal or obstructive renal disease. Apart from accelerated (malignant) hypertension, in which renal function can be impaired, the presence of non-malignant essential hypertension per se is not a major cause of advanced renal disease. High blood pressure, however, can accelerate the age related decline in glomerular filtration rate. Renovascular disease (renal artery stenosis) is a relatively uncommon cause of secondary hypertension, but it is potentially curable.

Regardless of the cause of renal impairment, hypertension considerably influences its progression. In people with diabetic and non-diabetic renal disease, two factors are important in preserving residual renal function: control of blood pressure and blockade of the renin-angiotensin system with angiotensin converting enzyme inhibitors or angiotensin receptor blockers.

The threshold for antihypertensive treatment in patients with persistent proteinuria or renal impairment is ≥140 mm Hg systolic blood pressure or ≥90 mm Hg diastolic blood pressure, or both. Optimal control of blood pressure is defined as <130/80 mm Hg, although reduction of blood pressure to <125/75 mm Hg may provide additional benefit in patients with chronic renal disease of any aetiology that is associated with proteinuria of ≥1 g/24 hours. Nonetheless, the recent African American study of kidney disease did not show that a lower target blood pressure (128/78 mm Hg) was better at preserving renal function in African Americans with non-diabetic chronic renal disease than less tight control of blood pressure (141/85 mm Hg).

Choice of therapy

Any drugs that are excreted by the kidney need to be given initially in small doses. This is particularly true for the angiotensin converting enzyme inhibitors and β blockers.

Angiotensin converting enzyme inhibitors have been shown to reduce microproteinuria and macroproteinuria, and some evidence suggests that they preserve renal function. Meta-analyses that examined the renoprotective effect of angiotensin converting enzyme inhibitors in patients with all forms of non-diabetic parenchymal renal disease confirmed a benefit of inhibition of angiotensin converting enzyme beyond that achieved with reductions in blood pressure, particularly in patients with overt proteinuria.

In patients with less advanced renal disease and those without overt proteinuria, blockade of the renin-angiotensin system may be less important in preventing the development or progression of renal impairment than control of blood pressure. Angiotensin converting enzyme inhibitors also may not be renoprotective beyond their antihypertensive effects in patients with polycystic kidney disease and hypertension.

The angiotensin converting enzyme inhibitors (and angiotensin receptor blockers) may also precipitate a deterioration in renal function in patients with bilateral renal artery stenosis. Caution is therefore needed in patients with renal failure who are taking diuretics, because the angiotensin converting enzyme inhibitors may produce large reductions in blood pressure if patients become dehydrated.

Data on the renoprotective effects of angiotensin receptor blockers in patients with chronic renal disease but without diabetes are limited. In the combination treatment of angiotensin II receptor blocker and angiotensin converting enzyme inhibitor in non-diabetic renal disease (COOPERATE) studies, the combination of an angiotensin receptor blocker and an angiotensin converting enzyme inhibitor was more effective at protecting renal survival than either drug alone.

Additional antihypertensive treatment is often needed and should include a thiazide diuretic or thiazide like diuretic.

Important clues that suggest renovascular disease

- Onset of hypertension before the age of 30 years
- Documented sudden onset of hypertension or sudden worsening of hypertension in middle age
- Accelerated (malignant) hypertension
- Resistant hypertension (to regimen of more than four drugs)
- Renal impairment of unknown cause
- Large elevation of serum creatinine, especially with marked reduction in blood pressure from treatment with angiotensin converting enzyme inhibitors or angiotensin receptor blockers (≥30% increase of creatinine)
- Peripheral vascular disease or severe generalised atherosclerotic disease
- Recurrent "flash" pulmonary oedema or heart failure with no obvious cause

---

Angiotensin converting enzyme inhibitors and serum levels of creatinine

- A small increase in serum levels of creatinine with angiotensin converting enzyme inhibitors is haemodynamic not nephrotoxic
- An increase of up to 30% is not an indication to stop angiotensin converting enzyme inhibitors
- If creatinine increases by >30%, angiotensin converting enzyme inhibitors should be withdrawn temporarily
- An increase of >30% can be caused by:
    —Hypotension
    —Dehydration
    —Bilateral renal artery stenosis
    —Non-steroidal anti-inflammatory drugs
    —Underlying chronic renal failure

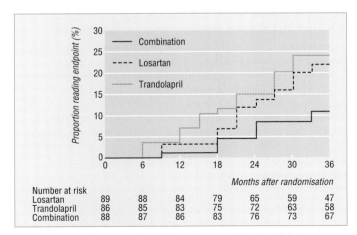

COOPERATE study: comparison of losartan, trandolapril and their combination in patients with diabetic renal disease (P = 0.02)

In patients with oedema and those with more advanced renal impairment (serum levels of creatinine > 200 μmol/l), thiazide diuretics and thiazide like diuretics are ineffective, and a loop diuretic (such as furosemide) should be used. Calcium channel blockers are effective and relatively safe in patients who have renal failure.

In patients with end stage renal failure, hypertension is common but can be controlled with dialysis. In anuric patients, salt and water restriction between dialyses sessions may be enough to control blood pressure, but drug treatment is often still needed. Patients with end stage renal failure are usually anaemic, and treatment with erythropoietin is usually initiated, although blood pressure may increase with this drug.

A high proportion of dialysis and renal transplant recipients develop hypertension, especially if they have received kidneys from donors with hypertension. Post-transplant hypertension in the early phase may be related to acute rejection or acute tubular necrosis that follows the ischaemic period, as well as some fluid overload if the patient was underdialysed before the operation. The use of corticosteroids as immunosuppressive agents can exacerbate fluid retention, and, in the long term, the use of cyclosporin A also may cause hypertension. Hypertension can develop in response to renin secretion from the patient's own atrophic kidneys, or atheromatous renal artery stenosis may affect the blood supply to the transplanted kidney. Good control of blood pressure is needed to preserve the function of the transplanted kidney.

Even mild persistent increases in urinary excretion of albumin (even below the threshold currently used to define microalbuminuria) and mild increases in serum levels of creatinine before antihypertensives are started are strong predictors of premature cardiovascular morbidity and mortality. Patients with end stage renal failure, and those on dialysis or after transplantation, have a particularly high incidence of atheromatous vascular disease, heart attacks, and strokes. Most patients with renal disease and treated hypertension are at substantial cardiovascular risk and will benefit from treatment with statins and aspirin.

Connective tissue disease

Rheumatoid arthritis, systemic lupus erythematosus, polyarteritis nodosa, and other connective tissue disorders are all associated with hypertension and an increased risk of cardiovascular disease. In some of these conditions, the hypertension is related to renal vasculitis. The tendency to develop hypertension is increased by the concomitant use of non-steroidal anti-inflammatory drugs, corticosteroids, gold treatment, and, in some cases, immunosuppressive drugs. In patients with progressive systemic sclerosis (scleroderma), hypertension is unusual unless the patient has evidence of renal involvement leading to progressive renal failure.

No clear guidance is available on the best antihypertensive drugs in these patients. In patients with scleroderma kidney, angiotensin converting enzyme inhibitors are frequently used. In other connective tissue diseases, most doctors opt for angiotensin converting enzyme inhibitors or calcium channel blockers, or both. β Blockers increase the tendency to develop Raynaud's syndrome and are best avoided. All patients with any connective tissue disease and hypertension, with or without overt renal involvement, need specialist referral.

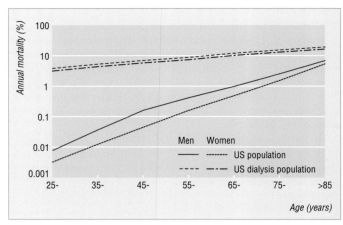

Cardiovascular mortality in patients on dialysis

Hypertension in patients after renal transplantation

- Found in about 50% of patients
- Related to cyclosporin and prednisolone
- Transplant renal artery stenosis
- Ischaemic damage during transfer
- Transplant rejection
- Recurrence of renal or systemic disease
- Hypertension from transplanted kidney
- Activation of the renin-angiotensin system
- Sodium and water retention

Hypertension and systemic lupus erythematosus

Patients with systemic lupus erythematosus	No of patients
All	656
With hypertension	200 (30.5%)

"In patients with systemic lupus erythematosus, hypertension is a potent independent risk factor for adverse renal outcomes and it also increases the risk of death"

The figure of hypertension in patients with diabetes is adapted from Krolewski AS, et al. *J Chron Dis* 1985;38:319–26. The figure of renin and sodium levels in patients with diabetes is adapted from Ferriss JB. *J Human Hypertens* 1991;5:245–54. The figure of the diabetic substudy of the losartan intervention for endpoint study is adapted from Lindholm LH, et al. *Lancet* 2002;359:1004–10. The figure of angiotensin converting enzyme inhibitors in patients with type 1 diabetes is adapted from Lewis EJ, et al. *N Engl J Med* 1993;329:1456–62. The figure of renal impairment as a risk factor for cardiovascular disease is adapted from Mann JF, et al. *Ann Intern Med* 2001;134:629–36. The box showing angiotensin converting enzyme inhibitors and serum levels of creatinine is adapted from Isles CG. *Clin Med JRCPL* 2002;2:195–200. The figure showing the results of the Cooperate trial is adapted from Nakao N, et al. *Lancet* 2003;361:117–24. The figure of cardiovascular mortality in patients on dialysis is adapted from Foley RN, et al. *Am J Kidney Dis* 1998;32:112–9. The table and comment on systemic lupus are adapted from Ginzler EM, et al. *J Rheumatol* 1993;20:1694–700.

12 Ethnicity and age

G Y H Lip, D G Beevers

Ethnic groups

Surveys in the United Kingdom and United States show that black people of African or African-Caribbean origin have higher levels of blood pressure and a greater prevalence of hypertension than white Caucasians. This greater burden of hypertension is associated with higher rates of renal failure, left ventricular hypertrophy, and stroke. By contrast, morbidity and mortality from coronary heart disease is lower in black people than in the white population.

In general, black patients are more sensitive to salt than white patients, and advice on salt restriction is particularly important. Much salt intake derives from processed foods rather than added salt, and education on restriction of salt intake should include dietary advice.

If drug treatment is needed, black people have different responses to antihypertensive drugs to white people and south Asian people. This is thought to be related to the low plasma levels of renin and angiotensin in black people. Blood pressure in black people responds better to thiazide or thiazide like diuretics and calcium channel blockers and poorly to β blockers, angiotensin converting enzyme inhibitors, and angiotensin receptor blockers. In a comparison of the calcium channel blocker verapamil and metoprolol in African-Caribbean patients with diabetes, metoprolol was no more effective than placebo but verapamil significantly reduced blood pressure.

These ethnic differences in response to antihypertensive treatment have significant implications for prognosis—for example, among the black (but not white) patients with hypertension in the antihypertensive and lipid lowering treatment to prevent heart attack trial study, stroke and coronary events were significantly more common among patients randomised to an angiotensin converting enzyme inhibitor than those randomised to chlortalidone. No differences in these endpoints were seen between those randomised to the thiazide or thiazide like diuretics and those randomised to the dihydropyridine calcium channel blocker amlodipine. These differences in outcome are largely explained by the fact that calcium channel blockers and thiazides are more effective at controlling blood pressure than angiotensin converting enzyme inhibitors.

The combination of diuretic treatment with angiotensin converting enzyme inhibitors, however, is as effective in black people as in white people. Alternatively, very high doses of β blockers or angiotensin converting enzyme inhibitors (or angiotensin receptor blockers) are needed to achieve the same degree of reduction in blood pressure. Nonetheless, in patients with renal impairment, an angiotensin converting enzyme inhibitor is still needed. For example, the African-American Study of Kidney Disease and Hypertension trial in African-American patients with renal impairment compared the angiotensin converting enzyme inhibitor ramipril with amlodipine and with the β blocker metoprolol. The trial was stopped prematurely because of worsening of renal failure in those randomised to amlodipine but not ramipril. The recent consensus statement of the Hypertension in African American Working Group emphasises the need to achieve effective reductions in blood pressure in tandem with protection against target organ damage.

Patients of south Asian origin with hypertension are at very high risk from coronary heart disease and diabetes mellitus. In

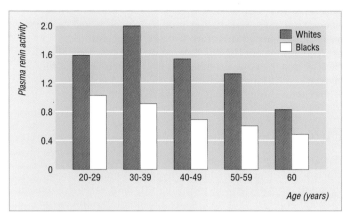

Plasma levels of renin in black and white patients with hypertension

> On average, only 10% of a person's salt intake is added in cooking or at the table. The rest is already present in foods

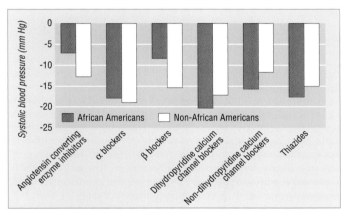

Ethnicity and response of systolic blood pressure to drugs

Hypertension in African American Working Group

- As initial monotherapy, the β blockers, angiotensin converting enzyme inhibitors, and angiotensin receptor blockers are less effective at reducing blood pressure in African Americans than white patients with hypertension because of the intrinsically low renin state in this ethnic group
- In contrast, thiazide diuretics and calcium channel blockers as monotherapy are much more effective at reducing blood pressure than other drug classes in African-Caribbean patients
- α Blockers should not be used as first line agents
- Although β blockers, angiotensin converting enzyme inhibitors, and angiotensin receptor blockers may be less effective as low dose monotherapy, the use of very large doses or the addition of a diuretic or a calcium channel blocker as a second agent would provide enough antihypertensive synergy to reduce blood pressure
- If "compelling indications" for prescribing β blockers, angiotensin converting enzyme inhibitors, or angiotensin receptor blockers are present in certain groups of patients with hypertension (such as "high risk" patients or those with target organ damage, including heart failure, coronary artery disease, or nephropathy), these indications should be applied equally to African-Caribbean patients

the United Kingdom, this population has higher mean levels of blood pressure and a higher prevalence of hypertension than the white population, as well as a higher risk of stroke. Essentially, no morbidity or mortality data from hypertension trials that relate to this population are available. In addition, no robust data are available to suggest that south Asian people respond differently to antihypertensive agents than white Caucasians. The thiazide diuretics, which can worsen glucose intolerance, should therefore be used with caution.

In people from the Far East, some epidemiological and clinical trial data are available. Of note, mean levels of blood pressure in Chinese people in the United Kingdom may be higher than those of people in mainland China.

Elderly people

Coronary heart disease and stroke are the major causes of mortality in elderly people, and hypertension is the most common treatable risk factor. A definition of ≥160/95 mm Hg means that more than half of the 12 million people in the United Kingdom older than 60 years are hypertensive. With a definition of ≥140/90 mm Hg, more than 70% of people will be hypertensive. In this patient group, isolated systolic hypertension is common, and, on an epidemiological basis, the degree of systolic hypertension is related more closely to stroke and coronary heart disease, even when underlying diastolic blood pressure is corrected for. An age related increase in pulse pressure is also seen.

Multiple measurements of blood pressure should be taken in elderly people to confirm the diagnosis of hypertension, as such patients tend to have greater variability in blood pressure. During the initial assessment, attention to symptoms and total cardiovascular risk should be checked. In addition, measurements of blood pressure with the patient in the seated and standing positions are needed to assess postural or orthostatic hypotension, which is more common in older people. If the latter is significant (for example, a decrease in systolic blood pressure with standing of ≥20 mm Hg with symptoms), antihypertensive treatment should be titrated to standing values of blood pressure. Ambulatory blood pressure measurement may be of particular value in identifying patterns of 24-hour blood pressure behaviour in the elderly (see Chapter 4). All elderly people with hypertension should be given lifestyle advice. In particular, a diet low in salt is more effective in elderly people than in younger patients.

The absolute benefits of antihypertensive treatment are much greater in elderly people with hypertension because of their increased absolute risk. Antihypertensive treatment may reduce dementia and impaired cognitive impairment associated with increasing age, as well as stroke and heart attacks.

In elderly patients, thiazide or thiazide like diuretics and calcium channel blockers are the drugs of first choice, as they reduce cardiovascular morbidity and mortality. β Blockers are not as effective as thiazide or thiazide like diuretics at reducing stroke deaths, coronary heart disease events, or all cause mortality in elderly people. Should diuretics or calcium channel blockers prove insufficient to control blood pressure, it is usual to add an ACE inhibitor or an angiotensin receptor blocker (ARB).

Very elderly people

In the very elderly (for example, those older than 80 years), the benefits of antihypertensive treatment have not yet been firmly established. Nonetheless, a meta-analysis of trials that included patients older than 80 years found that active treatment

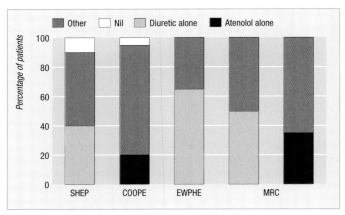

Antihypertensive drugs in elderly patients. (SHEP = systolic hypertension in the elderly; COOPE = Coope, J, et al. trial; EWPHE = European Working Party on high blood pressure in the elderly; MRC = Medical Research Council)

> The use of β blockers to treat hypertension in elderly people should be confined to specific indications, such as after myocardial infarction, angina, or systolic heart failure

> Most elderly people with hypertension need more than one antihypertensive to control their blood pressure

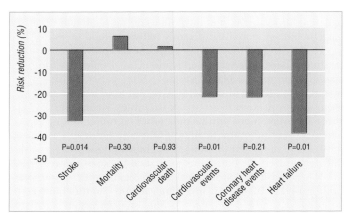

Meta-analysis of trial outcomes in patients > 80 years

> In the losartan intervention for endpoint trial, losartan was more effective than atenolol in reducing the risk of stroke and cardiovascular mortality in elderly people, including those with isolated systolic hypertension

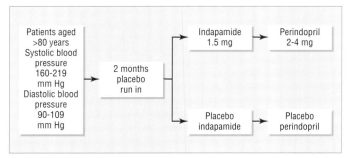

Trial design of the hypertension in the very elderly trial (HYVET)

reduced the incidence of stroke and heart failure (fatal and non-fatal) but a non-significant trend for an increase in all cause mortality was seen. One ongoing study—the hypertension in the very elderly trial—will assess the safety and efficacy of antihypertensive treatment in very elderly patients.

Hypertension in children

Hypertension is uncommon in children and, when present, indicates a great likelihood of underlying secondary causes, such as renal disease, coarctation, or vasculitis. A careful evaluation for secondary hypertension is therefore needed. In children younger than three years, measurement of blood pressure can be achieved only with Doppler flow equipment, and, of course, the appropriate sized cuff must be used in children of all ages. Children whose blood pressure is higher than the 90th percentile for their age need to be monitored; if blood pressure is higher than the 95th percentile, referral for further assessment and detailed investigation is mandatory.

Blood pressure increases sharply as children mature. Children who have higher blood pressures to start, especially obese children, tend to have a faster rise with advancing age. A recent analysis of two serially conducted cross sectional studies—third National Health and Nutrition Examination Survey (NHANES III) conducted in 1988–94 (n = 3496) and NHANES 1999–2000 (n = 2086)—showed that mean blood pressure has increased over the past decade among children and adolescents. This is partially attributable to an increased prevalence of obesity.

The Barker hypothesis (see chapter 3) suggests that the origin of adult essential hypertension may be found in childhood or even infancy. Babies with a low weight at birth have a greater risk of developing hypertension in later life.

To screen for hypertension in all children is not justifiable, but blood pressure should be measured in those who present with systemic illness, especially renal disease. When blood pressure is measured in children, phase V sounds may be difficult to hear, so the K4 diastolic Korotkoff sound may need to be recorded for infants and children aged 3–12 years and the K5 sound for adolescents aged 13–18 years. If K4 and K5 sounds are heard, both should still be documented.

As with the general management of hypertension, the approach to children initially should include non-pharmacological measures, such as weight reduction (if the child is obese), restriction of salt intake, and increased levels of exercise. Data from trials on drug treatments in this patient population are limited; however, β blockers, calcium antagonists, and α blockers are generally safe. Theoretically, the thiazide diuretics may have long term metabolic effects and perhaps should be avoided in children. The angiotensin converting enzyme inhibitors and angiotensin receptor blockers should also be used with care in patients with renal disease, but, on a long term basis, they probably are renoprotective in children as well as adults.

Hypertension in children

Age (years)	Mean blood pressure			
	Systolic		Diastolic	
	Normal mean	95th percentile	Normal mean	95th percentile
Birth–6 weeks	75	95	–	–
6 weeks–4 years	35	110	60	70
5–6	105	115	60	75
7–8	105	120	65	80
9–10	110	125	65	80
11–12	115	130	65	85
13–14	120	135	70	85
>14	–	140	–	90

Most common causes of sustained hypertension in children and adolescents

Age group	Cause
Newborn infants	Renal artery thrombosis
	Renal artery stenosis
	Congenital renal malformations
	Coarctation of the aorta
	Bronchopulmonary dysplasia
Infancy to 6 years	Renal parenchymal diseases
	Coarctation of the aorta
	Renal artery stenosis
6–10 years	Renal artery stenosis
	Renal parenchymal diseases
	Primary hypertension
Adolescence	Primary hypertension
	Renal parenchymal diseases
	Renal artery stenosis

The figure of plasma levels of renin in black and white patients with hypertension is adapted from Freis ED, et al. *Am J Med* 1983;74:1029–34. The figure of ethnicity and response of systolic blood pressure to drugs is adapted from Wu X, et al. *Am J Hypertens* 2005;18:935–42. The data in the figure showing antihypertensive drugs in the elderly are taken from: SHEP Cooperative Research Group. *JAMA* 1991;236:3255–64; Coope J, Warrender TS. *BMJ* 1986;293:1145–51; European Working Party on High Blood Pressure in the Elderly. *Lancet* 1985;1:1349–54; and Medical Research Council Working Party. *BMJ* 1992;304:405–12. The meta-analysis of patients > 80 years is adapted from Gueyffier F, et al. *Lancet* 1999;353:793–6. The trial design of the hypertension in the very elderly trial is reproduced with permission from Beckett NS, et al. *J Human Hypertens* 1999;13:839–40. Tables of hypertension in children and most common causes of sustained hypertension in children and adolescents are adapted from Second Task Force on Blood Pressure Control in Children. *Pediatrics* 1987;79:1–25.

13 Pregnancy and oral contraceptives

G Y H Lip, D G Beevers

Pregnancy

Hypertension in pregnancy is the most common cause of maternal death, with a risk of around 10 deaths per million pregnancies in the United Kingdom. Hypertension in pregnancy also is the most common cause of stillbirth and neonatal death. Hypertension occurs in 8–10% of pregnancies and may be the first sign of impending pre-eclampsia—a potentially more serious condition of the second half of pregnancy and puerperium.

Recent data from the United States show that pregnancy induced hypertension was the underlying cause in 16% of maternal deaths. More seriously, pre-eclampsia is responsible for one sixth of all maternal deaths and a doubling of perinatal mortality. Despite accurate figures on the effects of high blood pressure, its precise causes of hypertension in pregnancy are unknown; eclampsia has been referred to as a "disease of theories."

In pregnancy, diastolic blood pressure should be measured at the disappearance of sounds (phase V), not at muffling (phase IV), unless phase V goes to zero. Automated devices and devices for measuring ambulatory blood pressure have been validated for use in pregnancy.

In a survey of 6000 women in an unselected obstetric population in Oxford, 0.1% of women had blood pressure ≥160/100 mm Hg before the 20th week of pregnancy. This increased to 3.7% when the maximum antenatal reading at any stage of pregnancy was used. The threshold of ≥140/90 mm Hg was found in 2.0% of women in early pregnancy and 21.5% of women at some stage (usually very near to term). The combined frequency of pre-eclampsia and eclampsia varies between 1% and 6% depending on parity; the higher figure is seen in first pregnancies. In specialist hypertension obstetric clinics, rates are higher—11.9% and 16% for women with normal blood pressure and high blood pressure before pregnancy, respectively.

Most women with high blood pressure in early pregnancy (before 20 weeks' gestation) probably have pre-existing or chronic hypertension. This will often be "essential" hypertension, but clinical evaluation is needed, as secondary (usually renal hypertension) may present for the first time in pregnancy. Most women with high blood pressure in late pregnancy have pregnancy induced hypertension or pre-eclampsia, or this may even reflect hypertension that was undetected before the pregnancy and disguised by the decrease in blood pressure of early-mid pregnancy.

In the developed world, perinatal mortality is now approaching 10 per 1000 women, and just under half of these deaths are the result of high blood pressure. Furthermore, maternal mortality is low (about 50 deaths per million women) and about one fifth of these deaths can be attributed to all hypertensive diseases combined. In many cases of death as a result of eclampsia or pre-eclampsia (72% in one series), the care (diagnosis and management) was considered to have been substandard, with half of patients who died of eclampsia having had convulsions despite being admitted to obstetric wards.

Hypertensive syndromes in pregnancy

Several attempts have been made at classifying hypertension in pregnancy. None, however, is entirely satisfactory.

The Working Group of the American National Heart, Lung and Blood Institute classifies hypertension in pregnancy as:

Diagnoses during pregnancy

Pre-eclampsia
- Diagnosed on the basis of hypertension with proteinuria

Gestational and pregnancy induced hypertension
- Blood pressure >140 mm Hg systolic blood pressure or >90 mm Hg diastolic blood pressure after 20 weeks in a woman who was normotensive before 20 weeks' gestation
- Hypertension should be confirmed by two separate measurements

Proteinuria
- 300 mg/l protein or 30 mg/mmol creatinine in a random specimen or excretion of 300 mg/24 hours

Chronic hypertension
- Blood pressure 140/90 mm Hg before 20th week of pregnancy or, if only diagnosed during pregnancy, persisting six weeks after delivery

Pre-eclampsia superimposed on chronic hypertension
- Regarded as highly likely in women with hypertension alone who develop new proteinuria or in women with pre-existing hypertension and proteinuria who have sudden increases in blood pressure or proteinuria, thrombocytopenia, or increases in hepatocellular enzymes

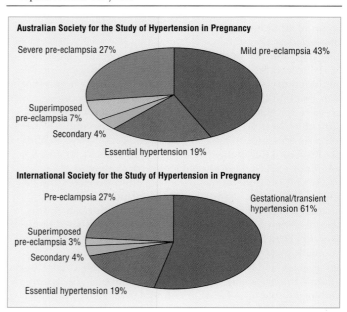

Comparison of two classifications of hypertensive syndromes of pregnancy in 1183 consecutive pregnancies

Problems with classification of hypertensive disorders of pregnancy

- Blood pressure is not measured before pregnancy in many women, and some may have had previous hypertension
- Blood pressure tends to settle in mid-pregnancy
- Differentiation between mild pre-eclampsia and less ominous rises in blood pressure in late pregnancy is difficult
- Whether increases in blood pressure in late pregnancy may proceed rapidly to severe pre-eclampsia cannot be predicted
- Many women are opting for later pregnancies and may have essential hypertension
- Ambulatory blood pressure monitoring is being used increasingly for the various forms of hypertension in pregnancy

- Chronic hypertension
- Pre-eclampsia
- Pre-eclampsia superimposed on chronic hypertension
- Gestational hypertension.

Gestational hypertension becomes transient hypertension of pregnancy if pre-eclampsia is not present at the time of delivery and blood pressure returns to normal by 12 weeks after birth and chronic hypertension if high levels persist.

Pre-existing hypertension

Probably the most benign category is pre-existing mild essential hypertension that is present before the 20th week of pregnancy, when the mother is assumed to have had pre-existing hypertension, although often no data are available. In these patients, blood pressure follows the normal pattern of pregnancy—it may fall during the first trimester and then increase again later in the pregnancy. This long term hypertension is not confined to or caused by pregnancy, but it may be noted for the first time during pregnancy, typically towards the end.

Of note, the usual "cause" of chronic hypertension is essential hypertension, but secondary causes of hypertension, although infrequent, may occur. About 5% of women of childbearing age have chronic pre-existing hypertension, which is usually mild. In women in their late 30 s and 40 s, this figure approaches 10%.

Pregnancy induced hypertension

Pregnancy induced hypertension usually develops after the 20th week of pregnancy and usually resolves within 10 days of delivery. This syndrome is common, occurring in up to 25% of first pregnancies, although it is less common (about 10%) in subsequent pregnancies. Some women who develop hypertension de novo early in the second half of pregnancy, however, are likely to progress to pre-eclampsia, with the development of proteinuria, thrombocytopenia, and oedema and the need for early delivery.

For diagnosis of pregnancy induced hypertension to be made, the blood pressure must be documented to be normal before and after pregnancy. The International Society for the Study of Hypertension in Pregnancy defines pregnancy induced hypertension as a single diastolic blood pressure (phase V) of 110 mm Hg or two readings of 90 mm Hg at least four hours apart after the 20th week of pregnancy. The National High Blood Pressure Education Program of the United States defines pregnancy induced hypertension as an increase >15 mm Hg in diastolic blood pressure or >30 mm Hg systolic blood pressure compared with readings taken in early pregnancy.

Pre-eclampsia

Pre-eclampsia is diagnosed with an increase in blood pressure >15 mm Hg diastolic or >30 mm Hg systolic from early pregnancy or a diastolic blood pressure of >90 mm Hg on two occasions four hours apart or >110 mm Hg on one occasion and proteinuria (proteinuria of 1+ is an indication for referral and >300 mg/24 hours is the criterion for diagnosis). About 30% of eclamptic convulsions occur in the absence of high blood pressure or proteinuria. Women with pre-eclampsia generally have no symptoms and can be detected only by routine screening. The most frequent symptoms are headache, visual disturbance (often "flashing lights"), vomiting, epigastric pain, and oedema. Women rarely present with a convulsion, but a first seizure in the second half of pregnancy with no other known cause is highly suggestive of eclampsia.

Pre-eclampsia is less common than pregnancy induced hypertension, occurring in about 5% of first pregnancies. Risk

Hypertension in pregnancy*

Variable	Blood pressure			
	Normal	Pregnancy induced hypertension	Pre-eclamptic toxaemia	Chronic hypertension
No (%) of women	625 (88.9)	55 (7.8)	12 (1.7)	11 (1.6)
Age (years)	23	25	23	28
Booking blood pressure (mm Hg)	107/64	114/68	112/66	131/91
Weight (kg)†	3.17	3.07	2.91	2.88
Ponderal index (kg/m²)†	24.6	23.1	23.8	23.3

*Data from 703 consecutive primiparous women at City Hospital, Birmingham.
†Adjusted for gestational age at delivery.

> Mild essential hypertension in pregnancy does not usually carry a bad prognosis for the mother or fetus

> Early treatment of mild essential hypertension does not convincingly prevent onset of pre-eclampsia

> Increasing evidence suggests that pregnancy induced (gestational) hypertension and pre-eclampsia may be broadly similar—the difference being a matter of severity

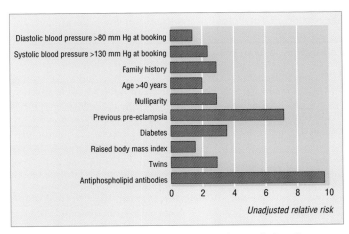

Risk factors for pre-eclampsia: systematic review of controlled studies

factors for pre-eclampsia include: first pregnancy, change of partner, previous pre-eclampsia, family history of pre-eclampsia, idiopathic hypertension, chronic renal disease, diabetes, systemic lupus erythematosus, multiple pregnancy, and obesity. Although the prevalence falls in subsequent pregnancies by the same father, pregnancies by different fathers are said to have the same rate as in primigravidas.

Pre-eclampsia is more common in women with diabetes and those of low socioeconomic status. The incidence of pre-eclampsia is increasing with advancing maternal age, but, paradoxically, the incidence is high in young teenage mothers. In addition, pre-eclampsia is associated with hydatiform mole and rhesus isoimmunisation.

The origins of pre-eclampsia relate to abnormalities of implantation of the placenta in the first trimester. Failure of development of the placental blood vessels leads to placental and fetal ischaemia in severe cases and eventually to placental infarctions. The fetus may have intrauterine growth retardation as it becomes hypoxic and ischaemic, and it may die. The circulating renin-angiotensin system is less activated than in normal pregnancies and, although disturbances of other vasoactive systems, such as angiogenic factors (vascular endothelial growth factor and its receptor, flt-1), the kallikrein-kinin system, and endothelin occur, the full importance of all of these changes is not understood fully. Although pre-eclampsia has its origins in the first half of pregnancy, it may not become clinically evident until 30 weeks' gestation.

Eclampsia

Full blown eclampsia is an obstetric emergency that has a very high risk for the mother and fetus. In addition to hypertension and proteinuria, often gross oedema is present. The more serious complications include cerebral oedema with convulsions, renal failure, pulmonary oedema, and disseminated intravascular coagulation. Fortunately, this condition is rare, occurring in one in 500 pregnancies.

Management of hypertension

Clinical management of hypertension in pregnancy aims to:

- Protect the mother from the effects of high blood pressure
- Prevent progression of the disease and occurrence of eclamptic convulsions
- Minimise risks to the fetus
- Deliver the fetus when the risk to the mother or fetus, if the pregnancy continues, outweighs the risks of delivery and prematurity.

Antihypertensive drugs are given to protect the mother—usually against the risk of stroke; however, they have only a limited effect on the progression of pregnancy induced hypertension or the development of pre-eclampsia. The precise benefits of pharmacological treatment for the fetus are also

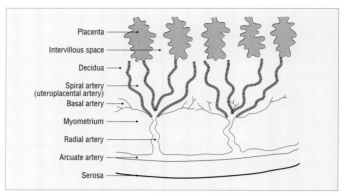

Blood supply to placenta in third trimester. Spiral arteries (hatched) have been converted to uteroplacental arteries from their origins from the radial arteries

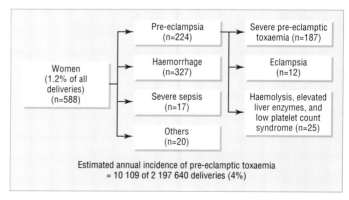

Blood supply to placenta in pre-eclampsia. Spiral arteries are not converted to uteroplacental arteries (solid outlines) or converted only in decidual segments (hatched outlines)

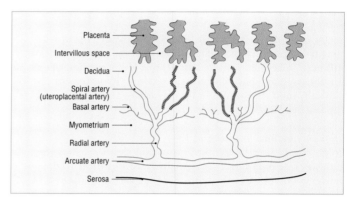

Severe obstetric morbidity in Southeast Thames survey

Laboratory tests in pregnant women with hypertension

Test	Rationale
Full blood count	Haemoconcentration is found in women with pre-eclampsia and is an indicator of severity Decreased platelet count suggests severe pre-eclampsia
Blood film	Microangiopathic haemolytic anaemia may occur in women with severe pre-eclampsia or eclampsia
Urinalysis	If dipstick proteinuria is ≥1, quantitative measurement of excretion of protein over 24 hour is needed Consider pregnant women with hypertension and proteinuria to have pre-eclampsia until proved otherwise

Serum levels:
  Uric acid
  Albumin
  Urea and creatinine
	
	High in women with pre-eclampsia or eclampsia
	May be low even with mild proteinuria, perhaps as a result of capillary leak or hepatic involvement in pre-eclampsia
	Usually low in pregnancy. "Normal" non-pregnancy levels may indicate renal impairment

Liver function tests	Levels of aspartate transaminase and alanine transaminase increase in women with HELLP syndrome*

*HELLP syndrome involves haemolysis, high levels of liver enzymes, and low levels of platelets.

controversial. One advantage is to prolong the pregnancy to allow the fetus to mature.

A meta-analysis of trials of antihypertensives in pregnancy suggests that the main benefits may be some reduction in the risk of progression to severe hypertension and fewer hospital admissions. Treatment certainly should be started if levels of blood pressure exceed 150–160 mm Hg systolic or 100–110 mm Hg diastolic. A drug that can be used safely in women who become pregnant should be chosen. Women with hypertension who plan pregnancy or become pregnant while taking antihypertensives should be switched to one of the drugs recommended for use during pregnancy. If possible, antihypertensives should be withdrawn under close follow up.

Many pregnant women may be mildly hypertensive (<150/100 mm Hg), but treatment may not be required, as these patients have a low absolute risk of developing pre-eclampsia. Women with essential hypertension who become pregnant are at risk of developing pre-eclampsia and intrauterine growth restriction. Such patients require close management, including frequent blood pressure checks, regular urinalysis, and assessment of fetal growth. Hospital referral is needed—preferably to a specialist antenatal hypertension clinic—in women with poor control of hypertension, new onset proteinuria, or suspicion of intrauterine growth restriction

The ultimate treatment of pregnancy induced hypertension and pre-eclampsia, as well as eclampsia, is delivery—certainly when the fetus is mature enough for the neonatal care facilities available. This option is needed in pregnant women with severe, persisting hypertension, in association with rapid weight gain, decreased creatinine clearance, significant proteinuria, evidence of fetal growth retardation, or the development of severe headache, papilloedema, hyperreflexia, scotoma, or right upper quadrant (hepatic) pain.

Post partum, blood pressure should continue to be monitored. Many women will need their previous anti-hypertensive drug regimen. Gestational hypertension and pre-eclampsia may lead to the future development of hypertension and an important increase in long term cardiovascular risk. Women with normotensive births have a lower probability of later hypertension.

Mothers who have had pre-eclampsia during a first pregnancy have a 7.5% risk of recurrence for their second pregnancy. Other causes of hypertension should be considered when a patient develops hypertension in pregnancy, especially if they have any unusual features or the hypertension is severe. A history of hypertension in pregnancy should not be a contraindication to oral contraceptives, but careful monitoring is essential. The developmental status of children born to women with pre-eclampsia is usually good.

At one time, strict bed rest was advocated once high blood pressure was established in a pregnant woman, but this approach was never shown to be of any value and is now discredited. Simple relaxation as an inpatient with a regular diet and no drugs can normalise blood pressure within five days in >80% of women admitted with mild pregnancy induced hypertension (although many subsequently become hypertensive again); however, no major difference in perinatal outcome is apparent with this approach. Sedatives and tranquillisers should be avoided.

Obesity in pregnancy can be associated with hypertension, with waist circumference up to 16 weeks' gestation predicting pregnancy induced hypertension. Mothers should be encouraged to avoid excessive weight gain in pregnancy, but they should not be advised to go on strict diets because of a detrimental effect on birth weight.

Comparison or outcome	Peto odds ratio (95% CI)	Number of trials
Maternal		
Severe hypertension	0.27 (0.14 to 0.53)	3
Additional antihypertensives	0.36 (0.23 to 0.57)	5
Admission during delivery	0.23 (0.07 to 0.70)	1
Proteinuria	0.70 (0.45 to 0.08)	6
Caesarean section	1.22 (0.81 to 1.82)	4
Abruption	0.42 (0.15 to 1.22)	3
Changed drugs owing to side effects	2.79 (0.39 to 20.04)	2
Perinatal		
Perinatal mortality	0.40 (0.12 to 1.32)	7
Prematurity	1.47 (0.75 to 2.88)	3
Small for gestational age infants	1.28 (0.69 to 2.36)	6
Neonatal hypoglycaemia	2.06 (0.41 to 10.29)	2
Low Apgar score (5 min <7)	0.90 (0.32 to 2.53)	3

Antihypertensive treatment in pregnancy for mild chronic hypertension

Comparison or outcome	Peto odds ratio (95% CI)	Number of trials
Maternal		
Severe hypertension	0.36 (0.26 to 0.49)	13
Additional antihypertensives	0.39 (0.26 to 0.59)	6
Admission during delivery	0.45 (0.30 to 0.67)	4
Proteinuria at delivery	0.67 (0.51 to 0.89)	12
Caesarean section	0.95 (0.76 to 1.20)	4
Abruption	2.50 (0.76 to 8.21)	7
Changed drugs owing to side effects	2.59 (0.93 to 7.20)	8
Maternal mortality	7.20 (0.14 to 363.10)	3
Perinatal		
Perinatal mortality	0.68 (0.36 to 1.25)	15
Prematurity	0.97 (0.72 to 1.31)	7
Small for gestational age infants	1.35 (0.96 to 1.88)	9
Admission to special care baby unit	1.04 (0.77 to 1.40)	7
Neonatal jaundice	0.53 (0.22 to 1.28)	2
Neonatal hypoglycaemia	0.76 (0.37 to 1.57)	3
Neonatal bradycardia	2.14 (1.09 to 4.20)	3
Low Apgar score (5 min <7)	0.56 (0.17 to 1.87)	3
Respiratory distress syndrome	0.27 (0.13 to 0.54)	5

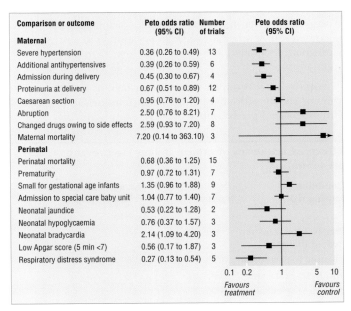

Antihypertensive treatment in late pregnancy

"Pregnancy seems to be a screening test for later chronic hypertension"

Leon Chesley, *Kidney Int* 1980;18:234–40

Restriction of salt intake is considered to be hazardous in pregnancy because it aggravates any plasma volume depletion and underlying renal impairment. Calcium supplements may reduce the incidence of pre-eclampsia and give a modest reduction in the incidence of high blood pressure, but no clear effect on other outcome measures is apparent.

Aspirin

Low doses of aspirin were previously advocated to prevent pre-eclampsia, although more recent evidence from trials has some inconsistencies because of the heterogeneous nature of the studies. One recent systematic review suggested a small protective effect. For example, early use of aspirin (150 mg/day) prevented fetal growth retardation and maternal proteinuria in women with fetal growth retardation, fetal death, or abruptio placentae in at least one previous pregnancy. In contrast, the Italian study of aspirin in pregnancy found that low doses of aspirin (50 mg/day) did not affect the clinical course or outcome of pregnancy. The large collaborative low dose aspirin study in pregnancy found that aspirin at a dose of 60 mg/day was associated with a non-significant reduction in the incidence of proteinuric pre-eclampsia, intrauterine growth retardation, stillbirth, or neonatal death.

The Australasian Society for the Study of Hypertension in Pregnancy recommends the use of prophylactic low doses of aspirin from early pregnancy in the following groups:

- Women with prior fetal loss after the first trimester, with placental insufficiency
- Women with severe fetal growth retardation in a preceding pregnancy either due to pre-eclampsia or unexplained causes
- Women with severe early-onset pre-eclampsia in a previous pregnancy requiring delivery at or before 32 weeks' gestation.

Aspirin is not routinely indicated for healthy nulliparous women, women with mild chronic hypertension and women with established pre-eclampsia

Effects of low doses of aspirin (60 mg) to prevent pre-eclampsia

Condition causing risk	No of women	No (%) of women who developed pre-eclampsia	
		Aspirin	Placebo
Pregestational insulin treated diabetes	471	18	22
Chronic hypertension	774	26	25
Multifetal gestation	688	12	16
Previous pre-eclampsia	606	17	19
Total	2539	18	20

None of these trends were significant. No differences in perinatal mortality, preterm birth, or infants small for gestational age.

Pre-eclampsia

Pre-eclampsia indicates urgent transfer to a specialised maternity unit with an adequate special care baby unit, together with antihypertensive and anticonvulsant treatment. Diazepam and magnesium sulphate help prevent fits and reduce levels of blood pressure.

The value of magnesium sulphate in the management of eclampsia is increasingly well established. Magnesium sulphate has the benefits of anticonvulsant and antihypertensive properties and is given intravenously or intramuscularly. It works quickly and has a nonsedative effect and wide safety margin. If toxicity occurs, an antidote exists in the form of calcium gluconate.

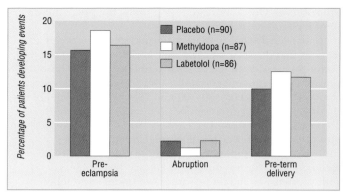

Randomisation trial of treatment of chronic hypertension in pregnancy

Drug therapy

Methyldopa

This remains the antihypertensive drug of choice during pregnancy, and its safety during pregnancy and post partum have been well characterised. Nonetheless, methyldopa can cause sedation, lethargy, and possibly postnatal depression.

Diuretics

These have not been recommended to treat hypertension in pregnancy, as they theoretically may cause a reduction in circulating volume and uteroplacental blood flow. Nonetheless, a meta-analysis of controlled trials of thiazide and thiazide like diuretics suggested a reduced incidence of pre-eclampsia. Certainly, no evidence shows that low dose thiazide diuretics are harmful in women with pre-existing hypertension.

Calcium channel blockers (especially long acting formulations of nifedipine)

These are sometimes used as second line drugs during pregnancy and are particularly useful in patients of African origin.

β Blockers

Increasing evidence suggests that atenolol and possibly labetolol cause intrauterine growth retardation, particularly if taken in early pregnancy. Their use is declining rapidly.

Labetolol

This was used widely as a second line agent, particularly for women with resistant hypertension in the third trimester. In small studies in women with severe hypertension, labetolol by intravenous infusion (20–160 mg/hour) or intermittent bolus (50–100 mg at 20–30 minute intervals) reduced blood pressure smoothly, although hypotension, oliguria, and bradycardia have been reported in neonates when fetal distress or hypoxia was also present.

α Blockers

These are probably safe, although the newer drugs, such as doxazosin and terazosin, have yet to undergo formal testing and may exacerbate urinary incontinence in women.

Angiotensin converting enzyme inhibitors and angiotensin receptor blockers

These drugs are contraindicated absolutely in pregnancy because of an association with congenital abnormalities, growth retardation, intrauterine death, oligohydramnios, and fetal anuria.

The Eclampsia Trial Collaborative Group has reported that magnesium reduces the risk of convulsions and has less maternal and neonatal morbidity than conventional anticonvulsants. The Magpie trial showed the efficacy of magnesium sulphate in halving the risk of mothers with pre-eclampsia progressing to eclampsia, with little or no risk to mother and baby. Prophylactic magnesium treatment has also been shown to reduce the risk of developing eclampsia.

Control of blood pressure is mandatory—usually with oral agents including methyldopa, labetolol, nifedipine, or hydralazine, or both. Labetolol and hydralazine may be given by infusion or injection.

Eclampsia

The first line of management is to control the seizures. Intravenous diazepam, usually 20–40 mg, is used. Occasionally, phenytoin is used to prevent recurrence of fits. Magnesium sulphate is a popular alternative anticonvulsant for use in women with eclampsia.

Intravenous hydralazine is a useful antihypertensive drug of first choice. It is given as a 5 mg bolus at intervals of 20 minutes or as an infusion of 25 mg in 500 ml of Hartman's solution, with the dose titrated against the woman's blood pressure. An alternative is intravenous labetolol. Patients should be admitted to well equipped and staffed obstetric units with adequate facilities for neonatal care.

If the woman is in labour, or induction is considered, an epidural anaesthetic may be helpful—to reduce the blood pressure and the tendency to fit by reducing the pain of uterine contractions. The ultimate treatment of eclampsia, however, is urgent delivery of the baby.

Oral contraceptive pill

Combined oral contraceptives increase blood pressure by an average of 5/3 mm Hg. Nonetheless, severe hypertension may be induced in a small number of women (1%). Blood pressure may increase rapidly many months or years after initial use of a combined oral contraceptive pill. Combined oral contraceptives are also associated with a higher risk of stroke and myocardial infarction. Progestogen only contraceptive pills do not increase blood pressure and are therefore recommended for women with hypertension who want to use oral contraception or those with hypertension induced by the combined oral contraceptive pill.

If a woman is found to have high blood pressure while taking an oral contraceptive pill, alternative methods of contraception should be considered. If these are unacceptable, it may be necessary to restart a progestogen only pill, and antihypertensive drugs may be needed. The hazards of an unplanned pregnancy in women are greater than the hazards of a small increase in blood pressure.

Hormone replacement therapy

Blood pressure increases with age and after the menopause, and the adjusted increase in blood pressure may be steeper after the menopause. The use of hormone replacement therapy does not cause blood pressure to increase, so it is not contraindicated in women with hypertension. Nonetheless, several large randomised trials have established that "opposed" hormone replacement therapy (containing oestrogen and progestogen) does not protect from cardiovascular disease or stroke of any type in the context of primary or secondary prevention.

Pre-eclampsia in primigravidae: risk of subsequent pre-eclampsia and later chronic hypertension

Variable	Pre-eclampsia in first pregnancy	Pregnancy with normal blood pressure
No of women	406	409
Pre-eclampsia in second (%)*** pregnancy	46.8	7.6
Later pre-eclampsia (%)**	20.7	7.7
Chronic hypertension (%)**	14.8	5.6

**P<0.001.
***P<0.0001.

> Women with chronic essential hypertension have a greatly increased risk of pre-eclampsia. Antihypertensive drugs do not reduce this risk. Such women have an increased risk of hypertension and its consequences in later life

> The precise mechanisms by which increases in blood pressure occur with the use of combined oral contraceptives are unclear, although an idiosyncratic effect may be present, as no subgroups particularly are susceptible

> Blood pressure should be measured before oral contraceptives are started and (at least) every six months after contraception begins

> Data on the relation of progestogen only pills to cardiovascular risk are limited and they are less effective contraceptives

The figure showing comparison of classifications of hypertensive syndromes of pregnancy is adapted from Brown MA, et al. *J Hypertens* 1997;15:1049–54. The table of hypertension in pregnancy is adapted from Perry KG, et al. *Br J Obstet Gynaecol* 1994;101:587. The figure showing risk factors for pre-eclampsia is adapted from Duckitt K, et al. *BMJ* 2006;330:565–7. The diagrams of blood supply to placenta in third trimester and in women with pre-eclampsia are adapted from Gerretsen G, et al. *Br J Obstet Gynaecol* 1981;88:876–81. The figure of obstetric morbidity in the Southeast Thames survey is adapted from Waterstone M, et al, *BMJ* 2001; 322: 1089–93. The figures for antihypertensive treatment in pregnancy for mild chronic hypertension and late pregnancy are adapted from Magee LA, et al. *BMJ* 1999;318:1332–6. The figure of treatment of chronic hypertension in pregnancy is adapted from Sibai BM, et al. *Am J Gynecol* 1990;162:960–6. The table on low doses of aspirin is adapted from Caritis S, et al. *N Engl J Med* 1998;70:1–5. The table of pre-eclampsia in primigravidae is adapted from Sibai BM, et al. *Am J Obstet Gynecol* 1986;155:1011–6.

Appendix: Cardiovascular risk prediction charts

How to use the cardiovascular disease risk prediction charts for primary prevention

The charts on the next page are for estimating cardiovascular disease risk (non-fatal myocardial infarction and stroke, coronary and stroke death, and new angina pectoris) for individuals who have not already developed coronary heart disease or other major atherosclerotic disease. They are an aid to making clinical decisions about how intensively to intervene on lifestyle and whether to use antihypertensive, lipid lowering and antiplatelet medication, but should not replace clinical judgment.

- The use of these charts is not appropriate for patients who have existing diseases that already put them at high risk such as:
  —Coronary heart disease or other major atherosclerotic disease
  —Familial hypercholesterolaemia or other inherited dyslipidaemias
  —Renal dysfunction including diabetic nephropathy
  —Type 1 and 2 diabetes mellitus
- The charts should not be used to decide whether to introduce antihypertensive medication when blood pressure is persistently at or above 160/100 mm Hg or when target organ damage due to hypertension is present. In both cases antihypertensive medication is recommended regardless of cardiovascular disease risk. Similarly the charts should not be used to decide whether to introduce lipid lowering medication when the ratio of serum total to high density lipoprotein cholesterol exceeds 7. Such medication is generally then indicated regardless of estimated cardiovascular disease risk.
- To estimate an individual's absolute 10 year risk of developing cardiovascular disease choose the chart for his or her gender, lifetime smoking status (smoker/non-smoker), and age. Within this square define the level of risk according to the point where the coordinates for systolic blood pressure and the ratio of total cholesterol to high density lipoprotein cholesterol meet. If no high density lipoprotein cholesterol result is available, then assume this is 1.00 mmol/l and the lipid scale can be used for total cholesterol alone.
- Higher risk individuals (areas in the darkest two shades of blue) are defined as those whose 10 year cardiovascular disease risk exceeds 20%, which is approximately equivalent to the coronary heart disease risk of >15% over the same period.
- The chart also assists in identifying individuals whose 10 year cardiovascular disease risk is moderately increased in the range 10–20% (blue area) and those in whom risk is lower than 10% over 10 years (light blue area).
- Smoking status should reflect lifetime exposure to tobacco and not simply tobacco use at the time of assessment. For example, those who have given up smoking within five years should be regarded as current smokers for the purposes of the charts.
- The initial blood pressure and the first random (non-fasting) total cholesterol and high density lipoprotein cholesterol can be used to estimate an individual's risk. However, the decision on using drug therapy should generally be based on repeat risk factor measurements over a period of time.

- Men and women do not reach the level of risk predicted by the charts for the three age bands until they reach the ages 49, 59, and 69 years respectively. The charts will overestimate current risk most in people under 40. Clinical judgement must be exercised in deciding on treatment in younger patients. However, it should be recognised that blood pressure and cholesterol tend to rise most and high density lipoprotein cholesterol to decline most in younger people already with adverse levels. Left untreated, their risk at the age 49 years is likely to be higher than the projected risk shown on the age under 50 years chart. From the age of 70 years the cardiovascular disease, especially for men, is usually ≥ 20% over 10 years and the charts will underestimate the true total cardiovascular disease risk.
- These charts (and all other currently available methods of cardiovascular disease risk prediction) are based on groups of people with untreated levels of blood pressure, total cholesterol, and high density lipoprotein cholesterol. In patients already receiving antihypertensive therapy in whom the decision is to be made about whether to introduce lipid-lowering medication, or vice versa, the charts can act as a guide. Unless recent pre-treatment risk factor values are available, it is generally safest to assume that cardiovascular disease risk is higher than that predicted by current levels of blood pressure or lipids on treatment.
- Cardiovascular disease risk is also higher than indicated in the charts for:
  —Those with a family history of premature cardiovascular disease or stroke (male first degree relatives aged <55 years and female first degree relatives aged <65 years) which increases the risk by a factor of approximately 1.5
  —Those with raised triglyceride levels (>1.7 mmol/l)
  —Women with premature menopause
  —Those who are not yet diabetic, but have impaired fasting glycaemia (6.1–6.9 mmol/l) or impaired glucose tolerance (2 hour glucose ≥ 7.8 mmol/l but <11.1 mmol/l in an oral glucose tolerance test)
- The charts have not been validated in ethnic minorities and in some may underestimate cardiovascular disease risk. For example, in people originating from the Indian subcontinent, it is safest to assume that the cardiovascular disease risk is higher than predicted from the charts (1.5 times).
- An individual can be shown on the chart the direction in which his or her risk of cardiovascular disease can be reduced by changing smoking status, blood pressure, or cholesterol, but it should be borne in mind that the estimate of risk is for a group of people with similar risk factors and that within the group there will be considerable variation in risk. It should also be pointed out in younger people that the estimated risk will generally not be reached before the age of 50, if their current blood pressure and lipid levels remain unchanged. The charts are primarily to assist in directing intervention to those who typically stand to benefit most.

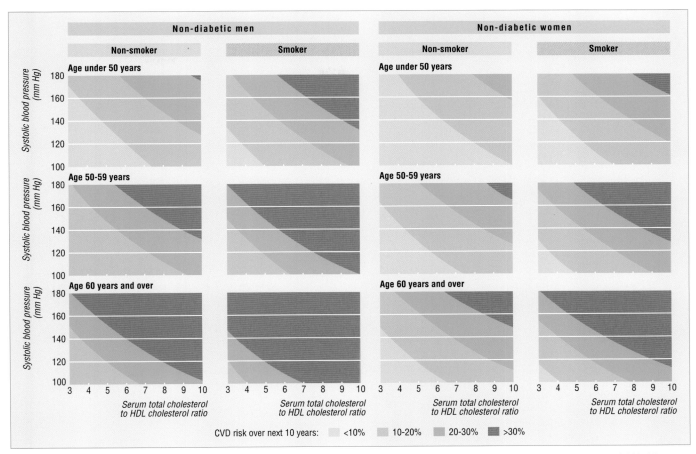

(HDL = high density lipoprotein). Adapted from *British National Formulary* 50, September 2005 (first published in *J Human Hypertens* 2004;18:139–85, copyright University of Manchester)

Index

Index

Index

Index